Praise for
the thyroid reset diet

"Important and indispensable. Everyone with thyroid disease should read *The Thyroid Reset Diet*. Dr. Alan Christianson makes the complexities of thyroid disease easy to understand and provides a straightforward plan that will enable most people with thyroid disease to either reverse it and/or resolve the symptoms caused by it. Highly recommended!"
—Steven Masley, MD, FAHA, FACN, CNS, bestselling author,
The 30-Day Heart Tune-Up

"Yes! You can reverse your thyroid disease symptoms. In *The Thyroid Reset Diet,* Dr. C. shows you how to fix your thyroid issues naturally. It's the most innovative treatment plan around and addresses the critical issue of how iodine really impacts your thyroid."
—JJ Virgin, New York Times bestselling author,
celebrity nutrition expert, and Fitness Hall of Famer

"Dr. Christianson's latest book is a science-backed deep dive into optimizing iodine levels for those with thyroid disease, and offers an easy-to-follow plan that makes this seemingly daunting lifestyle change doable. I highly recommend *The Thyroid Reset Diet* for anyone who is on their journey toward better days with hypothyroidism and Hashimoto's!"
—Izabella Wentz, PharmD, clinical pharmacist
and author of **Hashimoto's Protocol**

"If you are tired of complicated, restrictive diets, rituals, or cleanses that have not successfully restored your thyroid function, *The Thyroid Reset Diet* is the book for you. Dr. Alan Christianson expertly lays out an easy-to-follow plan allowing you to regulate your dietary iodine intake to optimize thyroid function, thereby preventing the need for lifelong thyroid medication."

—Brittany Bohinc Henderson, MD, ECNU, board-certified endocrinologist, Charleston Thyroid Center

"Naturopathic physician Dr. Alan Christianson has written the first book that focuses on what may be the main culprit behind Hashimoto's: excessive iodine intake. He offers new insights and a holistic treatment plan, including dozens of tasty recipes that can be used with all dietary preferences. A must read!"

—Anthony Youn, MD, FACS, America's Holistic Plastic Surgeon and bestselling author of **The Age Fix**

"All of Dr. Christianson's books are required reading for my patients, and *The Thyroid Reset Diet* is no exception. Dr. C. is a true leader in the world of hormonal health, and *The Thyroid Reset Diet* is a mandatory piece of the library of any person who wants wonderful thyroid health."

—Shawn Tassone, MD, PhD, author of **The Hormone Balance Bible**

the thyroid RESET diet

the thyroid RESET diet

Reverse Hypothyroidism and Hashimoto's Symptoms with a Proven Iodine-Balancing Plan

Alan Christianson, NMD

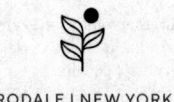

RODALE | NEW YORK

Rodale Books
An imprint of Random House
A division of Penguin Random House LLC
1745 Broadway, New York, NY 10019
RodaleBooks.com | RandomHouseBooks.com
penguinrandomhouse.com

2025 Rodale Trade Paperback Edition

Copyright © 2021 by Alan Christianson, NMD

The material in this book is for informational purposes only and is not intended as a substitute for the advice and care of your physician. As with all new diet and nutrition regimens, the program described in this book should be followed only after first consulting with your physician to make sure it is appropriate to your individual circumstances. The author and publisher expressly disclaim responsibility for any adverse effects that may result from the use or application of the information contained in this book.

Penguin Random House values and supports copyright. Copyright fuels creativity, encourages diverse voices, promotes free speech, and creates a vibrant culture. Thank you for buying an authorized edition of this book and for complying with copyright laws by not reproducing, scanning, or distributing any part of it in any form without permission. You are supporting writers and allowing Penguin Random House to continue to publish books for every reader. Please note that no part of this book may be used or reproduced in any manner for the purpose of training artificial intelligence technologies or systems.

Rodale & Plant with colophon is a registered trademark of Penguin Random House LLC.

Originally published in hardcover in the United States by Rodale, an imprint of Random House, a division of Penguin Random House LLC, in 2021.

LIBRARY OF CONGRESS CATALOGING-IN-PUBLICATION DATA
Names: Christianson, Alan, author.
Title: The thyroid reset diet / Alan Christianson, NMD.
Description: New York: Rodale Books, [2021] | Includes bibliographical references and index.
Identifiers: LCCN 2020036658 | ISBN 9780593137062 (hardcover) | ISBN 9780593137086 (paperback) | ISBN 9780593137079 (ebook)
Subjects: LCSH: Thyroid gland—Diseases—Alternative treatment. | Thyroid gland—Diseases—Diet therapy.
Classification: LCC RC655 .C477 2021 | DDC 616.4/40654—dc23
LC record available at https://lccn.loc.gov/2020036658

Printed in the United States of America on acid-free paper

9 8 7 6 5 4 3 2 1

BOOK TEAM: Production editor: Annette Szlachta-McGinn • Managing editor: Allison Fox • Production manager: Angela McNally

The authorized representative in the EU for product safety and compliance is Penguin Random House Ireland, Morrison Chambers, 32 Nassau Street, Dublin D02 YH68, Ireland. https://eu-contact.penguin.ie.

I dedicate this book to you, the reader. People with thyroid disease need better options. This book is a brand-new option and I'm excited to share it with you. No matter how long you've struggled, don't give up. You can feel better. You deserve nothing less.

Thanks go first to my wife, Kirin. Honey, thank you for your patience despite all the time I spent working on this project. You always encourage me to keep at it when you know the results might help someone. I love you.

Thanks go to my children, Celestina and Ryan. Celestina, thank you for inspiring me to be creative and independent. Ryan, thank you for inpiring me to think at a deeper level and to get through the tough parts of a project.

Thanks to our doctors and our team at DrC online and Integrative Health. It is a great feeling to know that you you are there to help me scale what I do well and to make up for what I can't do well. None of this work would be possible without you.

Contents

	Introduction	11
Chapter One	**The Thyroid Dilemma**	19
Chapter Two	**Your Thyroid Might Surprise You**	33
Chapter Three	**The #1 Cause of Thyroid Disease**	45
Chapter Four	**Invisible Iodine**	57
Chapter Five	**Thyroid Reset Diet**	81
Chapter Six	**The Maintenance Phase**	111
Chapter Seven	**Food Lists and Meal Assembly**	127
Chapter Eight	**Recipes and Meal Plans**	151
	The 28-Day Meal Plan	152
	Shakes	157
	Other Breakfasts	167
	Salads, Bowls, and Wraps	179
	Soups and Stews	194
	Main Courses	203
	Sides, Dressings, and Dips	226
	Desserts	238
Chapter Nine	**FAQ**	241
	In Closing	255
	Shopping Lists	257
	Notes	263
	Acknowledgments	275
	Index	277

Introduction

People with thyroid disease struggle with symptoms like fatigue, mood changes, weight gain, and hair loss. They try everything to feel better—medications, supplements, dietary changes. Yet most never hear about the one change that may help them the most. I'm happy to tell you that there is a new way forward—one that doesn't include debilitating symptoms and constant doctor visits.

A new chapter is emerging for thyroid health, and someone needs to tell it. In 2007, doctors celebrated the 100th anniversary of Dr. Hiroko Hashimoto's original paper that defined thyroid disease. He discovered that most thyroid disease was caused by the immune system attacking the gland. We call it chronic autoimmune hypothyroidism, or Hashimoto's disease, because of his work. Along with the recognition of a century's passage came hard questions: What do we have to show for the last hundred years? How far have we come to understand this condition and in helping people feel better?

Those answers have been sobering. Too many people are still undiagnosed, and surveys have shown that of those who are diagnosed, too few have had their symptoms resolved. This realization spurred a flurry of new information, and much of it was original research. This new information included insights gleaned through careful new analysis of existing research. Many have thought that our changing diets are somehow to blame. They are right, but not in the ways we expected.

Results have shown that regulating iodine intake could reverse thyroid disease, even in those who have severe thyroid disease. These studies were dramatic, and other scientists soon replicated them. Some showed complete disease reversal in as many as 80 percent of the participants. Never has any other treatment had such an effect on thyroid disease. My goal in writing this book is to help you join that lucky 80 percent.

We now know that thyroid disease is more reversible than previously thought. We also know that we are exposed to iodine from more sources and in higher amounts than originally thought. The amount of iodine in many common foods has been rapidly increasing, unbeknownst to many. Indeed, the connection between iodine and thyroid disease is fascinating. It turns out that iodine is unlike any other nutrient, in many ways.

Most nutrients are used by the body for producing countless reactions. Yet iodine is used almost solely in the thyroid, and only for the purpose of making thyroid hormones. Normally, the blood carries as much of most nutrients as the tissues need to function. But iodine has to be concentrated in the thyroid up to 100-fold above typical blood levels. For most nutrients, it is easy to get enough of what we need without getting too much; there is a wide range between the lowest effective amount and the lowest toxic dose. With iodine, though, that safe range is far narrower. Finally, most nutrients are found in foods in predictable amounts, yet iodine can vary wildly from batch to batch—in the same food.

How can a nutrient cause a disease that affects the only part of our body that needs it? It can be a hard concept to grasp.

Iodine is one of the nutrients your thyroid needs to build thyroid hormones. When your body gets a tiny amount of iodine, everything works as it should. Imagine the size of a single uncooked lentil; that is how much iodine your thyroid needs for an entire year.

Your thyroid simply cannot handle too much iodine. Indeed, the mass of iodine equal to 1½ lentils per year could easily cause thyroid disease. In fact, it is so powerful that even the right amount of iodine can cause problems if it's not consumed in regular amounts over time. Further, your thyroid can get rid of excess iodine only by producing thyroid hormones. Yet at the same time, excess iodine slows down the production of those thyroid hormones. Hence, consuming too much iodine can slow the thyroid. And like iodine intake, thyroid hormones cannot fluctuate significantly without having consequences.

With such narrow parameters for healthy thyroid function, humans have experienced thyroid disease for as long as recorded history. But it's getting worse. In past decades, people in many parts of the world were found to be iodine deficient. We've now overcorrected for that deficiency, with many people getting far more iodine than they need—and yet they are unaware of the problem. This consumption of excess iodine is showing up in the growing numbers of people with thyroid disease. Based on age and ethnicity, from 30 to 40 percent of American adults are consuming unsafe levels of iodine. Many of them are lucky enough to tolerate it; those who can't tolerate it get thyroid disease.

If you are among the millions of people with an unsafe iodine intake, that could be why thyroid disease is holding you back. So, the Thyroid Reset Diet may be your answer. The diet described in this book is a new approach to the problem. In a word, numerous clinical trials have shown that careful iodine reduction can successfully reverse thyroid disease and eliminate its symptoms. This book is the first time that approach has been made available to the public, and it comes in the form of a healthy diet that does not restrict food categories. Think of this book as mountains of that new research shaped into a simple action plan just for you. Indeed, this diet can help your thyroid heal, and then restore it to good function. If you were recently diagnosed with hypothyroidism and/or Hashimoto's thyroiditis, there is a good chance that this diet plan could reverse your illness.

Thankfully, researchers have recognized that thyroid disease is a growing epidemic. They have launched countless new clinical trials, while at the same time investing thousands of hours in reanalysis of past studies. Among the top clues that led these researchers to this action were the observations made from the effects of low-iodine diets, which doctors were already using to increase the effectiveness of certain medical procedures.

The thyroid is the one part of the body that concentrates iodine. Based on this principle, doctors have used radioactive iodine to make an image that they can examine for diagnosis. For instance, they look at thyroid tissue to determine if it is somewhere it does not belong or they check if there are growths inside the thyroid that are not absorbing iodine like the surrounding tissues. Further, doctors give much higher doses of radioactive iodine to slow a person's overactive thyroid. In both cases, the radioactive iodine procedure works best when the thyroid is "hungry" for that iodine. These patients go on low-iodine diets for several weeks so that their thyroid will take in as much of the radioactive iodine as possible before the scan.

Researchers have discovered that many people see their thyroid function improve while they are preparing for the scan. Many doctors observed this patient response and they wondered if it was just a coincidence or if it might be a useful phenomenon. It seems the preparatory low-iodine diet might help guide other treatments. So, researchers launched clinical trials in which they carefully monitored the effects of a low-iodine diet. People with significant thyroid disease were put on low-iodine diets and they were compared to others with the same degree of thyroid disease who were not on that special diet. Neither group was given thyroid medication, or any other treatment.

The studies all yielded the same results. Nearly everyone who was *not* on the diet stayed just as sick or got worse. Yet of those who *were* on the low-iodine diet, roughly 80 percent had normal thyroid function within as little as three months. Nearly all who did not improve either did not avoid iodine as recommended, or did improve, but were not cured just yet.[1] It would seem likely that, given a few more months, they would have been fine, too.

I do not believe that this diet approach will help everyone with thyroid disease, but in accord with the published studies, nearly every person who was able to lower his or her iodine intake saw dramatic improvements in thyroid function.

Our knowledge about iodine grew on other fronts during this time, as well. For example, researchers found evidence of how excess iodine causes thyroid disease on a molecular level. It turns out that the human thyroid is good at making do with just tiny amounts of iodine; it concentrates every speck it gets from the bloodstream, storing it inside itself. Yet, as noted earlier, the thyroid can easily get overloaded with iodine, and a chronic excess of iodine slows the thyroid, damages it, and causes the immune system to attack it.[2]

In fact, we saw clear evidence of the iodine-thyroid connection in countries that were newly fortifying their salt with iodine. For example, Denmark fortified its salt with iodine beginning in the year 2000, but they had started tracking their population in 1997, suspecting that rates of thyroid disease could change. And change they did. For the following sixteen years that they studied, thyroid disease of all types rose year after year.

ISN'T IODINE GOOD FOR US?

Most people do not think much about iodine. Of those who do, they are more likely to believe the dangers of getting too little. For instance, iodine deficiency used to be a scourge. In the mid-twentieth century, it was found that a billion people were at risk for poor brain development, owing to iodine deficiency. As recently as 1990, people in only a handful of countries were getting enough iodine, and 112 countries were categorized by the World Health Organization (WHO) as "severely iodine deficient."

So, global organizations banded together to eradicate this problem. They were successful, and the iodine status of the world's countries changed over the next twenty-four years. By 2014, the number of nations considered severely iodine deficient plummeted to zero. This reversal in iodine deficiency was viewed as a clear win for the world. But as we now know, iodine has a narrower range of safety than any other nutrient. In short, it is easy to get too much iodine.

Around this same time, iodine was becoming a more popular ingredient with industrial food producers, and simultaneously more people were eating more processed food. The WHO recognizes that iodine levels considered more than adequate or excessive can trigger thyroid disease. There are now are over fifty countries that have more than adequate or excessive iodine. The United States is one of them.[3] The following chart compares iodine deficiency between 1990 and 2014.

	1990	2014
Number of nations with severe iodine deficiency	112	0
Number of nations with above necessary or excessive iodine	0	52

This global spike in iodine consumption exactly parallels the skyrocketing increase in thyroid diseases such as hypothyroidism, Hashimoto's, and thyroid cancer, the latter instance of which has risen roughly sevenfold during this time frame.

Correlation by itself does not prove causation, of course, but it does when the correlation converges with other lines of evidence. In the following chapters, I share details on how multiple lines of evidence have all converged to show that excess iodine truly is the culprit when it comes to thyroid disease.

Yes, there are other factors associated with thyroid disease, such as age, gender, and genetics. Yet iodine is the only major factor that can be changed, and it has been proven to be worth changing. The truth is, most thyroid disease is driven by simple choices that you have control over—once you are aware of them. These changes are

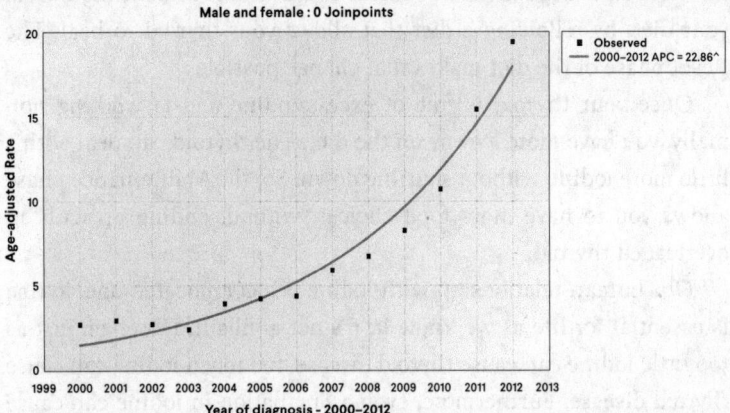

Source: Du L, Wang Y, Sun X, et al. Thyroid Cancer: Trends in Incidence, Mortality and Clinical-Pathological Patterns in Zhejiang Province, Southeast China. *BMC Cancer.* 2018;18(1):1–9. doi:10.1186/s12885-018-4081-7

much easier to make than those found in many popular (and less effective) diets.

There are invisible sources of iodine sneaking into peoples' diets, even as they try so hard to eat carefully. Invisible sources of iodine can also sneak in from cosmetics. These hidden sources combine with the obvious sources of iodine that are in supplements and medications. To make matters worse, many functional medicine practitioners give megadose iodine supplements to people with thyroid disease.

In 2004, I started getting countless patients who had never had thyroid disease until they started taking megadose iodine supplements. Yes, the thyroid needs iodine. It seems logical to think that if the thyroid is not working, extra iodine would get it going again. The basic idea was plausible, but the more I studied the matter, the more it became clear that those megadoses of iodine were much more likely to make things worse.

The good news is that all is not lost. You should not and do not need to avoid all sources of iodine. Most people will obtain better thyroid function if they simply lower their iodine intake enough to let their thyroid clear out its excess. In *The Thyroid Reset Diet*, you'll learn how to locate those invisible sources of iodine and remove them from your diet, by following a diet that allows your thyroid to heal. The Reset phase of the diet makes that change possible.

Once your thyroid is free of excess iodine and is working normally, you have more leeway on the diet. The thyroid can deal with a little more iodine without shutting down. So, the Maintenance phase allows you to have more food choices, without ending up with an overloaded thyroid.

Our human relationship with iodine is a complicated one. Iodine is essential for life as we know it; it's not a villain. However, just as too little iodine can cause thyroid disease, too much iodine can cause thyroid disease. Furthermore, even a fluctuation in iodine can cause thyroid disease.

Healthy thyroid function comes from giving your body the right amount of iodine regularly. If you have had thyroid disease for some time and are taking thyroid medication, this approach may lower your need for that medication, or even eliminate it. But you will need personalized guidance on this path, and later chapters here offer suggestions and resources.

In this book, I share with you an exciting story. You will learn why thyroid disease happens, why it is on the rise, and how you can reverse it. I ask you to keep an open mind. Much of the new research I present may run contrary to what you now know about thyroid disease. It certainly has surprised me.

Please know that thyroid disease is serious, and it can act differently in different people. Along with this dietary plan, you'll need personalized guidance from a thyroid specialist you can trust. Use this book as a tool in conjunction with the care of your doctor.

The most important thing I have learned is the first that I can share with you: thyroid disease *can* get better. Thank you for giving me a chance to tell you how. Let's dive in!

Chapter One

The Thyroid Dilemma

This book will show you how to reset your thyroid—usually in as little as a few months. For many, a "reset" means the symptoms clear up. The fatigue, stubborn weight, and brain fog will disappear, or the hair loss will stop. For many, it also means that the thyroid may no longer need outside help. With the right guidance, you may be able to safely stop thyroid medication.

After decades of helping people deal with thyroid disease, I have seen how absolutely devastating this condition can be. Indeed, it can get in the way of everything that matters in life. But we now know that thyroid disease is a process, not a permanent condition. Thyroid disease needs a surplus of iodine to keep going, and once that excess iodine is eliminated, the thyroid can heal.

My patients have tried all sorts of diets to help with their thyroid disease; some have cut out gluten, dairy, processed grains, eggs, or animal foods, only to find that nothing works consistently. It turns out that these diets often cut out many, but not all, of the high-iodine foods. But the truth is that iodine can hide out successfully even in healthy diets. It can even sneak its way in through cosmetics and supplements. The Thyroid Reset Diet will help you hone in on the true invisible sources of iodine, while opening plenty of options from different food categories.

We've made more progress in learning about iodine and the thyroid in the last several years than in the last five decades, and this book is the first to show that careful regulation of iodine can reverse thyroid disease. *The Thyroid Reset Diet* provides simple action steps to help your thyroid heal. You won't need to eliminate certain food categories; instead, you'll choose low-iodine alternatives within those categories.

We're overdue for a new perspective on thyroid disease, because more people have it than ever before, and the conventional approach is just not working. Estimates are that as many as one in four women will eventually develop thyroid disease. For every person who knows he or she has thyroid disease, another one or two already have it but have not yet been diagnosed.[1]

Most thyroid conditions are caused by autoimmune disease. The immune system goes awry and attacks the thyroid, leaving it too damaged to work. Incidences of autoimmune thyroid disease have been increasing faster than nearly any other chronic condition, and its most common form is Hashimoto's thyroiditis. In the United States, Hashimoto's thyroiditis was once a rarity. But for women in their late thirties, its rates have gone up over twenty-five-fold since the early twentieth century.[2]

These trends also show up for other types of thyroid disease. The American Thyroid Association recently stated: "The incidence of thyroid cancer has increased dramatically during the past three decades, and it is now the fastest-growing cancer in women."[3] If conventional medicine lacks the explanations for this phenomenon, it should least be able to manage the symptoms—but that's not the case.

The American Thyroid Association recently asked over 12,000 people with thyroid disease how well their thyroid treatment was working. The respondents were between 31 and 61 years of age, and 96 percent of them were women. The results were abysmal.

- Fewer than 7 percent of respondents were "very satisfied" with their treatment.
- Over 70 percent changed doctors multiple times. In fact, 15 percent of the respondents had seen six or more different doctors.
- Over 80 percent of patients exclaimed that there was a strong need for new treatments.[4]

Current treatments do not work as well as they could because they are based on faulty principles. They assume that the core problem is a lack of thyroid hormone. In truth, the lack of hormone is often the body's response to too much iodine.

Thankfully, thyroid care can have a better outcome. I introduce you to Jennifer, who came to me as a new client because of her extreme tiredness.

Jennifer: A Typical Story

When we met, Jennifer started our talk by apologizing that her story was complicated. I encouraged her to take her time and tell me everything. I asked her to start by telling me when her symptoms had started and how her life had changed since then.

About four years ago, at her daughter's seventh birthday party, Jennifer remembered thinking to herself that life was surprisingly good. They had moved not too long ago and were settled in and happy. Things were falling into place for her. Her daughter had lots of new friends at her school, her career was in a good place, and she felt happier and more fit than she had for some time.

That was just before things started to change.

She started to get tired for no reason. Her workday seemed to drag on. Little things that she would have ignored in the past started to get to her. The inevitable extra requests or interruptions started to overwhelm her. She found herself wanting to eat out more often to avoid the effort of cooking and she had little patience for her family.

Everyone has the occasional off day, but she realized that this was something more than that. At first, she attributed the fatigue to having too much on her plate. Jennifer started taking her vitamins regularly, but they did not help.

Deciding it was about time, she found a primary care doctor through her insurance. After Jennifer told the doctor about her fatigue, he ran some tests. When the results came back, he told her that her thyroid was low and that she should take a prescription for it. The prescription was for a thyroid hormone called T4. He explained that Jennifer's thyroid was making too little T4 and the prescription would make up for the difference.

He told her that she had thyroid disease. It often happens for no clear reason, but it is more common when family members have it. When she asked what she should expect, he said that most people feel normal within a few months of starting the medication, but some do not get better. It seemed odd to Jennifer, because no one in her family had thyroid disease. Nonetheless, she started taking her prescription. She was relieved to have an explanation and a plan of action.

For the first few weeks, it seemed she was back to normal. But after three months, she was just as tired as she was when she first started taking it. She also noticed a new symptom—her weight started creeping up. The doctor suggested that Jennifer see an endocrinologist for further help.

The endocrinologist did additional blood tests and an ultrasound study of her thyroid. When the results were available, she told Jennifer that she had Hashimoto's thyroiditis. Jennifer learned that this diagnosis meant her thyroid was underactive because her immune system was attacking it. She explained that the treatment her primary care doctor started Jennifer on often worked, but some people with Hashimoto's needed to take an additional medication called T3 to feel better.

Jennifer started the second medication and felt much better within the first few days. It was hard to get her hopes up because that was just how it started last time. At the end of the second month, the benefits of the second medication wore off. The endocrinologist made several more adjustments over the next year. Some seemed to help at first. Some did not. Either way, Jennifer was still too tired.

By this point, it was starting to show. She was too tired to drive her daughter to after-school activities, she no longer had the energy for her exercise classes, and she was no longer as present as she used to be at work. Nor was she losing the weight she had gained. A friend suggested she see a functional medicine practitioner for another opinion.

Jennifer's functional medicine practitioner had been taught that autoimmune thyroid disease was caused by gluten or an iodine deficiency. He advised her to take a megadose iodine supplement and go on a diet that avoided gluten, other grains, dairy, and nightshade vegetables, like tomatoes.

The diet was hard to do, but she made it work. She felt fine the first few weeks and was pleased to see that she was losing a few pounds. And then things fell apart.

She had been tired before, but now she was debilitated. Not only could she not work, but she also could not stand up without feeling dizzy. Her endocrinologist retested her and found out that her thyroid was lower than ever, even with the medication. It was as if she was not taking any medicine at all.

The doctor suggested a higher dose and a retest in three months.

Jennifer's confidence had been shaken. She felt worse than ever. Her experience showed that raising the dose never gave her lasting relief. She did not feel like she could hold out for much longer without a major change, which brought her to my office. After Jennifer told me her story, I asked about her prior diet and asked to see her recent medications and supplements. The lab tests showed that she was getting too much iodine from somewhere.

I explained to her that her doctors were right. She had thyroid disease because of an autoimmune attack. She was surprised when I told her that the biggest single reason for autoimmune thyroid disease was too much iodine. When your body has too much iodine, it fights against thyroid hormones. That is why it is common to initially feel better on thyroid treatment, only to have the improvement lapse. At first, the extra hormone makes up for the lack. Within a few weeks, the body starts fighting harder and the old symptoms come back.

As we unraveled her story, it seemed that the first signs of fatigue may have been early thyroid disease, or they could have been just from her being overextended. By the time the primary care doctor tested her, Jennifer's thyroid was slowing, but there were no signs of autoimmune disease. By then, she was taking extra vitamins.

A recent analysis of over-the-counter vitamins showed that they often had two to three times more iodine than the label stated. Most people can safely ingest between 50 and 200 mcg of iodine per day from all sources. Jennifer's vitamins had three times that much, or more. The iodine in her vitamins, plus what was already in her diet, had likely started slowing her thyroid. The megadose of iodine is what caused her medication to quit working altogether. I explained to Jennifer that when an emergency room doctor needs to immediately stop an overactive thyroid to save someone's life, he or she uses megadose iodine.

Nothing stops your thyroid faster than a megadose of iodine. Even though she stopped taking it a month ago, her iodine levels were still dangerously elevated.

Jennifer was initially concerned when I told her that I did not want to change her thyroid medication. I asked here to keep it where it was and retest it in a month. I was confident that it would work differently once we corrected her iodine levels.

To do that, I needed to get Jennifer's daily iodine intake low enough so that her thyroid had a chance to get rid of all the iodine that had built up inside it.

I asked her to stop all remaining supplements that had iodine. I told her that some personal-care products like face creams and cosmetics can have too much iodine. I gave her a list of ingredients to look for and asked her to check her products when she got home.

Then, we talked about the Thyroid Reset Diet. She was already avoiding high-iodine foods like eggs, dairy products, and processed grains. She was happy to hear that non-dairy substitutes were safe, as were egg whites, whole grains, and home-baked products. Since she did not eat much seafood and rarely ate sea vegetables (which can be huge culprits of excess iodine), the only real change was trading sea salt for kosher salt. Considering the dietary changes she had already gone through, that was an easy request.

When I saw her after the first month, her demeanor was much improved. She said that within the first few weeks, she started getting her energy back. It seemed so natural that she did not notice it until she found herself energetically participating in her exercise class. She was still taking the last prescription from her endocrinologist and her blood levels showed that now it was working fine.

Eight weeks later, Jennifer called with a new symptom: her heart had started racing. Now that it was free of the iodine overload, her thyroid was starting to work by itself again. Since it was producing more thyroid hormone, the prescription now contained too much for her. I lowered her prescription and kept monitoring. We kept reducing her medicine over the course of eight months.

By then, Jennifer was back to her old energy levels and taking the smallest possible dose of thyroid medication. She no longer had signs of autoimmune thyroid disease, and her weight was back within a few pounds of where she liked. She felt confident that by continuing her healthy habits, it would be back to ideal shortly.

I had her switch to the Maintenance phase of the Thyroid Reset Diet. This change meant that she could have some dairy foods and egg yolks on occasion. It also meant that she had more options for seafood. She still needed a tiny dose of thyroid medicine, but since she felt so much better, taking a single pill was not a big deal.

Most people with thyroid disease are in the same situation as Jennifer.

So, if excess iodine is to blame, where is the extra iodine coming from? As we saw from Jennifer's story, iodine can hide in dairy, processed foods, commercially baked goods, supplements, and skin and hair products.

More of our food is heavily processed than ever before, and that can mean more iodine, as well. The FDA's *Total Diet Study* found that when comparing foods from 1991 with those in 2011, researchers found that the amount of iodine increased in twenty-three of the top twenty-five foods. Some of these foods in 2011 contain three times as much iodine as they had twenty years earlier.[5]

Iodine is added to foods because it has many properties that are useful in industrial applications. First, iodine works a lot like bleach. Both are halide chemicals, and therefore they make effective industrial sanitizers. Second, iodine can form gels that bind with water. That is why carrageenan is so widely used in processed foods and cosmetics—it helps control the texture.

Another problem is that iodine is such a volatile chemical; it is hard to control during the production cycle. That is why supplements with iodine, and iodine added to salt, show little consistency from batch to batch. These fluctuations by themselves are harmful to the thyroid, even if the average amount over time is reasonable.[6] In many ways, total iodine intake can reflect how much of the diet comes from processed foods.

Along with foods, iodine has become a real problem in supplements.

First, nearly all multivitamins have iodine. Most adults do not need additional iodine, and quality control in these vitamins is terrible. A large study analyzed the iodine content from a group of over 120 popular vitamins. Not a single product had the amount of iodine that was stated on the label. Many had two to four times more iodine than was stated.

Apart from the iodine in multivitamins, products that feature high doses of iodine have become popular. Countless people take iodine supplements based on outdated medical advice. They are hoping to improve their thyroid function, but sadly that makes it much worse. As mentioned, when the thyroid gland is exposed to too much iodine, it can lower its absorption of iodine, but this reduction can be kept up only for a few weeks. Once the gland starts to absorb iodine again, the extra iodine builds up in the gland. Thankfully, the body does have protective mechanisms in place.

Rather than let the extra iodine cause runaway production of thyroid hormones, the body slows down the thyroid. In doing so, it lowers the rate of thyroid hormone production in the thyroid, but it also makes the rest of the body less responsive to the thyroid hormones. That is why people with thyroid disease often do not feel better, even when they take thyroid hormone medications.

For some, these protective mechanisms do not work well enough. Their thyroid becomes overactive, and they go on to develop iodine-induced hyperthyroidism. For others, this slowdown is too heavy-handed. Their thyroid shuts down completely and they develop iodine-induced hypothyroidism. Even if the thyroid can slow itself down to the right degree, the extra iodine is still harmful. It forms free radicals, which damage its cells. This ongoing damage can alert the immune system, leading to iodine-induced autoimmune thyroid disease.

The good news is that most of these issues stop once the gland can get rid of the extra iodine.

THE THYROID RESET DIET

The Thyroid Reset Diet lowers your iodine levels so that the excess iodine can be cleared out. This gives your thyroid a chance to work as it should, and it restores your body's responsiveness to the thyroid hormones.

If you have Hashimoto's thyroiditis or hypothyroidism and are not on thyroid medications, the diet often takes three to six months to restore thyroid function. If you are on thyroid medication, it may take three to nine months longer because your team will need to gently reduce your medication.

Feeling better is often the first sign of your thyroid starting to reset. The most common symptoms of thyroid disease are fatigue, stubborn weight, hair loss, and forgetfulness. When the cells of the muscles, fat, hair follicles, and brain respond to thyroid hormones again, you'll get your energy, your memory, and your body back. Because this first change takes place inside the cells, it can happen before the blood levels change.

When the thyroid starts to recover, the blood tests show it. In the case of the study I mentioned in the introduction, the TSH scores of the participants went from an average of 14 IU/mL down to well within normal (normal is 0.4–4.5 IU/mL).

The Thyroid Reset Diet recommends that you test your thyroid regularly after starting the diet. Regular tests and appropriate adjustments of your medication not only keep you safe but also give your thyroid the best chance to recover. If you take too much medication, the extra amount may crowd your thyroid and slow its recovery. Yet if you lower the medication too quickly, the sudden demand on your newly recovered thyroid may overwhelm it.

Removing high-iodine foods from your diet is the backbone of the plan. Thankfully, these restricted foods are contained within a small set of food categories, and each of these food categories has plenty of low-iodine options. For example, egg yolks are high in iodine, but egg whites have none. Nearly any dish that is made with whole eggs can be made with egg whites. Commercially baked bread often has unsafe amounts of iodine, but it is easy to make bread that has nearly none. Dairy products often have high amounts of iodine, but some can be used in small amounts and there are many non-dairy substitutes that are safe to use.

This Thyroid Reset Diet is more complete than a typical low-iodine diet. Low-iodine diets were designed to be used only for one to three weeks before an iodine uptake procedure. They do not have to be simple or nutritionally sound, because no one is expected to be on them for any length of time. The Thyroid Reset Diet regulates iodine, but does so with more considerations. It is carefully constructed to be nutritionally complete, allowing it to be safely followed for a long term. It also incorporates other nutritional factors known to improve thyroid health, such as selenium and zinc and appropriate distributions of fats, proteins, and carbohydrates.

It is also distinct from past thyroid diets in that it does not require you to restrict entire food groups. If you follow a specific diet for other health reasons, you are welcome to continue. You can easily make the diet your own. I've given suggestions in this book to help you thrive regardless of whether you are just a healthier eater, gluten-free, vegan, paleo, or autoimmune paleo.

HOW DOES THE THYROID RESET DIET WORK?

All foods are organized into a simple system of Green Light, Yellow Light, and Red Light foods. Green Light foods have under 10 mcg of iodine per serving, Yellow Light foods may have up to 50 mcg per serving, and Red Light foods often have over 50 mcg of iodine per serving.

You start with the Reset phase, during which you're free to eat any of the Green Light foods while avoiding all Yellow Light and Red Light foods. The reset provides just under 100 mcg of iodine daily, along with all the necessary vitamins and minerals. It also supplies abundant amounts of healthy fats, good carbs, and essential proteins. Once your thyroid is well nourished and given a chance to get rid of the extra iodine, it can start to heal. The Reset phase gives you simple guidelines you can use to build your meals. If you like more structure, you can also follow the 28-Day Meal Plan (see page 152) with shopping lists (see page 258) and recipes (see Chapter Eight).

As your symptoms improve and your thyroid starts to work better, you will be able to see clear changes in your tests. This book will guide you regarding what to test and what to look for. The process works best when a health professional provides specific feedback. Indeed, if you are on thyroid medications, professional care is essential. Later chapters will help you put together your thyroid team, if you do not already have one.

Once your thyroid function stabilizes, you will be guided into the Maintenance phase. Here you will have even more food options. All the Green Light foods are still allowed, and you will still avoid the Red Light foods as much as possible. You have the option of adding up to two servings of any Yellow Light food per day.

The Maintenance phase will keep you between 50 and 200 mcg of iodine per day. The Maintenance phase also has simple guidelines and meal suggestions. All the recipes in the Reset phase are fine to use during the Maintenance phase. I also offer suggestions on how you could modify them now that you have more leeway.

Arianna: A Return to Normal

Arianna was 36 and was diagnosed with hypothyroidism three years ago. She went to see her doctor because she knew that something was wrong. Her weight had shot up 23 pounds in the last year. It had never been an issue in the past. She was also exhausted all the time. She had two young kids, and it broke my heart to hear her say that she was "too tired to be a good mom."

As frustrated as she was with her symptoms, she hated the idea of being stuck on medication even more. She felt there had to be another option.

She went gluten-free, and then tried a version of the autoimmune paleo diet. It seemed to help some people she met on social media, but her thyroid levels did not improve. She connected with my work on social media and decided to try the Thyroid Reset Diet. She was encouraged because it was completely different from (and easier than) anything she had tried.

Her prior diet did have her eliminate dairy and processed grains, but after reading the Thyroid Reset Diet guidelines, she realized that she was likely getting extra iodine from kelp supplements, iodized sea salt, and egg yolks.

She reached out to me after six weeks on a diet. Her thyroid levels were now normal for the first time in over three years. She was no longer tired and she felt like her old self. Her weight was not yet back to target, but it was starting to go down.

She plans to stay on the Reset phase until her thyroid levels are optimal, and her weight is within 5 pounds of her goal. She now feels that her kids will be able to have their mom back. She also knows some simple ways to adjust the family diet to lower her daughters' risk of developing thyroid disease. Her story shows that this does not have to be something that defines the rest of your life.

Arianna's timeline was not unusual. Most people take the first week to get into the hang of the new diet. From there, it takes another three to six weeks for measurable changes to show up on your blood levels.

From the clinical trials, roughly 80 percent of people show a clear shift in how much hormone their thyroid gland is making within the first twenty-eight days. They are not always back to normal by then, but they are at least showing progress. The vast majority show normal thyroid function within the first three months. Of those who do not, most of them see normal thyroid function within the first six months.

The exciting point is that the thyroid gland is more resilient than we used to think. Like the rest of the body, it is constantly renewing itself and growing new cells. As the conditions that gave rise to the disease are no longer present, the new cells work better. As the old cells gradually get replaced, you get a brand-new thyroid. For many, this is the same as a brand-new chance at life.

We now have a clearer understanding of why thyroid disease happens. This understanding explains why thyroid disease is on the increase. We have clear mechanisms of action, population studies, and placebo-controlled clinical trials that are all lining up. We have solutions that can prevent and even reverse the disease.

First, it helps to have a better understanding of the marvel that we call the human thyroid.

Chapter Two

Your Thyroid Might Surprise You

The thyroid gland is unlike any other gland in the body—no other gland controls so many functions with such microscopic amounts of hormone. Moreover, no other part of the body is as dependent on a single nutrient.

None of the typical ways in which nutrients work in the body apply to the thyroid and its relationship with iodine. As you learn the basics of how your thyroid works, you will come to understand how the tiniest deviations in iodine intake can lead to thyroid disease.

THYROID BASICS

The thyroid is a tiny lump of tissue in the neck. With a little imagination, you might think it almost looks like a butterfly. It sits below the Adam's apple and above the collarbone, just beneath the skin. You might be surprised at how small the thyroid is; it's about the size of two or three stacked credit cards. When it is healthy, you should not be able to see it or feel it.

The sole purpose of the thyroid is to make thyroid hormones. Hormones are chemicals the body releases into the bloodstream as a means of relaying signals from one part of the body to another. The purpose of hormones is to get the cells to alter what they are already doing or to do something new.

Cells are far too tiny to see or hear, but they can taste. Imagine you had a group of workers who were always sipping some water. They shared the same water cooler, and their boss added flavors to the water cooler to send messages. If the water tasted like citrus, that might mean things were going well. If it tasted like banana, that could mean it was time to break for lunch. If the water was spicy, that could mean the building was on fire and they should drop everything and run. The thyroid hormones are one of the several hormonal flavors that our cells taste. These hormones cause the cells to work harder and make more connective tissue. They also regulate other hormones, and they control how fast signals from nerves move throughout the body.

These changes to the cells are normally subtle. They work behind the scenes to keep all the body's systems operating as they should. Yet because these processes are critical, there are catastrophic consequences when the level of thyroid hormones are off. Those tiny chemical glitches can add up to dramatic effects that we see and feel.

For example, when our metabolic rate is low, everything we do is more sluggish. We can gain weight for no reason and it won't go away, despite intense efforts. Energy levels can run lower; fatigue sets in early in the day and exercise feels like a chore. The brain moves slowly, as well. Words can be hard to find, and even the simplest decisions feel like too much work. There can also be a buildup of fluids, resulting in swelling in the ankles or legs, along with a feeling of being bloated.

Because proteins are not formed correctly, the body has a hard time making repairs. Hair loss may speed up and hair growth may come to a standstill. The skin can feel dry and irritated. Nails become brittle and ridged. Muscles and tendons may feel sore for no obvious reason. The most minor exercise can create soreness and unexpected injuries.

When thyroid hormones decrease, additional symptoms appear because other hormones are being poorly regulated. For instance, any symptoms of perimenopause or menopause can become much worse. Periods can be heavy or irregular. Mood swings of PMS can be much more intense.

The most striking thing is that all this can result when there are differences in only the tiniest quantities of thyroid hormones. Imagine dropping 1 teaspoon of vanilla extract into an Olympic-sized pool. Those pools are half the length of a football field, just about as wide, and 6 feet deep. That teaspoon of vanilla mixed into a giant pool of water is almost exactly how diluted the thyroid hormones are in the human bloodstream. Yet your cells can "taste" them, so the exact amounts are critical.

If you added ½ teaspoon to the pool instead of 1 teaspoon, your cells would die. If you poured in 1 tablespoon instead of 1 teaspoon, your cells would overwork and collapse. I hope this gives you a sense of how potent the thyroid hormones are.

The main thyroid hormone is called T_4, also called levothyroxine. It is a thyroid protein with four iodine atoms stuck to it. The thyroid also makes T_3, also called triiodothyronine, which has one fewer iodine atom. There are other hormones that are also important, like T_2, reverse T_3, tiatricol, and many others. Some of these hormones are made directly by the thyroid, while others are made by the body from thyroid hormones. For simplicity's sake, I will refer to this entire group collectively as the thyroid hormones.

We use a measuring unit called a microgram (mcg) to describe things in such small quantities. A microgram is exceedingly small. For example, a gram is about the weight of a paper clip, and a milligram is a thousandth of a gram—about the mass of a grain of salt. That is, a microgram is a thousandth of a milligram, or a millionth of a gram. To give meaning to these comparisons, consider that the mass of a microgram to the mass of a paper clip is like the mass of a paper clip to the mass of an adult Holstein cow!

So, how exactly does your thyroid work and what do all these "T" hormones do?

TALE OF THE "Ts"

Consider that the thyroid can be lazy; it only works when the boss tells it to. The minute the boss stops giving orders, the thyroid goofs off.

Our first "T" word is the TSH, or thyroid stimulating hormone. It is the signal that the boss—otherwise known as the pituitary gland—sends to the thyroid. So, when the thyroid is not giving the body enough hormones, the pituitary sends some TSH to make it work harder. The less active the thyroid is, the more TSH is released by the pituitary gland. An underactive thyroid leads to *hypo*thyroidism. That is, low thyroid = higher TSH.

Also, there are times when the thyroid makes too much hormone. Normally, if the pituitary gland lowers production of TSH, the thyroid slows down and things are fine. But sometimes this does not work. In some cases, the thyroid gets its wires crossed and keeps on releasing hormones. Or, someone might be on a dose of thyroid medication that's more than they need. An excess of thyroid hormone is called *hyper*thyroidism. In these cases, the TSH first drops below range, then drops as low as possible—under 0.01. That is, high thyroid = low TSH.

The next "T" is for thyroglobulin (Tg), the main protein from which thyroid hormones are made. If a thyroid hormone is a car, then thyroglobulin is the chassis and iodine atoms are the wheels that go on in the final stages of assembly. Thyroglobulin is made inside thyroid follicles. Iodine is pushed into the follicle by a special pump called the sodium iodide symporter, or NIS for short.

Each day, your thyroid will use 50 to 200 mcg of iodine to make the thyroid hormones.[1] Because so little is needed, the thyroid can store a two- to three-month supply of iodine. That is why it may take a few months to clear out the excess iodine when there is too much. Just to put things into perspective, your lifetime supply of iodine could be carried in a teaspoon![2]

Iodine will stick to thyroglobulin by itself, but an enzyme called thyroid peroxidase, or TPO, makes it stick faster. When there's too much iodine, things go awry. The follicles are damaged, and the immune system can start to attack the thyroglobulin and/or the thyroid peroxidase. This is the start of autoimmune thyroid disease. A healthy person may have 8 to 10 iodine atoms on each molecule of thyroglobulin; when there is excess iodine, there may be as many as 60 on each molecule.

The last "Ts" are for the thyroid hormones themselves. T4 is a piece of a thyroglobulin molecule with 4 iodine atoms. T3 has 3 iodine atoms. T4, T3, and T2 are the active thyroid hormones; they all have effects on the body's metabolic rate and the production of proteins, with some subtle differences between them. Further, your brain controls how much hormone is released from your thyroid. After the hormones enter your bloodstream, the rest of your body adjusts how these hormones are converted and how quickly they are eliminated. Your liver takes the lead in this process.

As important as the thyroid hormones are, and as carefully as they are regulated, it is hard to imagine how this process can go wrong. But it can.

WHEN THYROID LEVELS ARE OFF

We have known for well over a century that things go wrong when thyroid hormones are catastrophically too low or too high. Imagine instead of 1 teaspoon of vanilla, the pool gets only a drop or, conversely, maybe it gets an entire bottle. These symptoms are specific, and doctors can recognize the conditions easily.

But what about when they are off by much smaller amounts?

The thyroid gland is composed of thyroid cells, and each cell lives only for a few months. There are always some old cells dying off and new cells stepping up to take their place. When the death and growth of cells is stable, the thyroid stays the same size. When the body needs more thyroid hormones, the brain tells the thyroid cells to get to work. The balance between new cell growth and old cell death needs to be perfect, though. If not in balance, the thyroid enlarges, shrinks, or gets lumpy. Such growth problems are the cause of nodules, goiters, and thyroid cancer.

The other way things can go wrong is if the thyroid produces the wrong amount of hormones, leading to either hyperthyroidism or hypothyroidism.

HYPERTHYROIDISM

With too much thyroid hormones in the system, the entire body becomes overstimulated. Symptoms include a racing heart, a sense of panic, trembling hands, and insomnia. If untreated, hyperthyroidism can cause fatal heart damage or long-term harm to the brain and bones.

The two most common causes of hyperthyroidism are Graves' disease and toxic nodular goiter. Like all versions of thyroid disease, both conditions are more common when iodine intake is not optimal. However, it is not clear whether a reduction in iodine can reverse the hyperthyroidism after it has started.

Hyperthyroidism demands urgent treatment. The acute dangers of the disease make it less amenable to lifestyle treatment only. Oddly enough, hyperthyroidism is more apt to reverse with appropriate medical treatment than hypothyroidism. For these reasons, we won't be focusing on hyperthyroidism here.

HYPOTHYROIDISM

Most people who have chronic thyroid disease have hypothyroidism, Hashimoto's thyroiditis, or both. These are also types of thyroid disease that respond best to the Thyroid Reset Diet. Therefore, from here on, when I refer to thyroid disease, I am referring to hypothyroidism and Hashimoto's thyroiditis.

Diagnostic standards define hypothyroidism as an elevated TSH score, a low T4 score, and the presence of classic hypothyroid symptoms. Most doctors consider a TSH elevated when it is above 4.5 IU/mL.

Thyroid symptoms are any combination of symptoms with no other explanation. These include fatigue, weight gain, hair loss, dry skin, dysmenorrhea, irritable bowel syndrome (IBS), bloating, muscular pain, difficulty swallowing, pressure in the throat, or voice changes.

Hypothyroidism can be brought about by surgery to remove the thyroid or as a reaction to a medication. But when hypothyroidism seems to happen on its own, the culprit is nearly always an autoimmune reaction against the thyroid.

HASHIMOTO'S THYROIDITIS

Hashimoto's thyroiditis is a condition in which the immune system attacks the thyroid. If the attack is significant enough, the thyroid sustains too much damage to make as much hormone as the body needs.

Doctors know someone has Hashimoto's thyroiditis when they can see presence of thyroid-attacking antibodies like anti-thyroid peroxidase (anti-TPO) and anti-thyroglobulin (anti-Tg) on their blood tests or the signs of autoimmune damage on an ultrasound. Ultrasound findings with Hashimoto's often includes numerous pockets of broken-down tissue, high amounts of blood flow, and extra blood vessels.

Hashimoto's is the most common cause of hypothyroidism. And most people who have Hashimoto's either also have hypothyroidism or will eventually develop it.

In some lucky cases, doctors detect the thyroid disease at the earliest stages; but usually, it's not diagnosed until symptoms show up.

SYMPTOMS OF THYROID DISEASE

Thyroid disease causes such distinct and widespread symptoms because the thyroid hormones play a critical role in so many of the body's processes, as you can see from the list that follows:

Symptoms of Altered Metabolism

- Coldness, especially of the extremities
- Depression/anxiety
- Fatigue
- Fluid retention, especially under the eyes
- Weight gain

Symptoms of Poor Tissue Repair

- Brittle nails
- Difficulty swallowing
- Dry skin
- Hair loss
- Hoarse voice
- Joint pain
- Tendonitis

Symptoms of Irregular Nerve Impulses

- Constipation
- Diarrhea
- Dizziness
- Muscle cramps
- Muscle pain
- Poor coordination
- Poor memory
- Tremors

Symptoms of Poor Hormone Regulation

- Headaches
- Hot flashes
- Insomnia
- Irregular periods
- Night sweats
- PMS
- Poor libido

***

Thyroid disease symptoms normally appear because the body has the wrong amount of thyroid hormones present. However, recent data do suggest that the inflammation from an autoimmune disease may cause symptoms even before the thyroid slows down. Thankfully, the Thyroid Reset Diet can help with both autoimmunity and thyroid hormone levels by reversing the main cause of both—iodine excess.

Some symptoms, like weight gain and fatigue, are typical of a deficiency in thyroid hormones, and others, like palpitations and anxiety, are caused by an overabundance. Yet doctors who treat thyroid disease know that nearly any symptom can be caused by either too much or too little thyroid hormones.

All of this happens because thyroid hormones work together with other hormones in the body, much like instruments in a symphony. If the thyroid levels are not right, the cells may not properly respond to other hormones. This poor response is the reason why abnormal thyroid levels can affect the regularity of menstrual cycles and fertility. Even if estrogen and progesterone are there, the cells will not respond to them properly if the thyroid is off.

Our nerves react to stimuli that we are not even aware of, as well as the signals that make us move. The wrong amount of thyroid hormone can cause a resting hand to tremble. Involuntary nerves, like those in the intestinal tract, are also affected. Thyroid hormones control peristalsis, or the movement of the intestines. Without the correct amount of hormones, gas, bloating, constipation, or diarrhea can be the result.

Of course, the biggest cluster of nerves is in the brain. Even small changes in thyroid levels can cause dramatic shifts in mood and mental state. Along with anxiety and depression, thyroid disease can cause symptoms that are often mistaken for psychosis or bipolar disorder.[3] The symptoms can be many, but some are more predictive of thyroid disease than others.

THYROID SYMPTOM SURVEY

The following symptom survey has been clinically validated and used in numerous research studies, including our own. These specific questions will help you measure your well-being and evaluate whether things are getting better or worse.

It is good to have a baseline reading of your current state so that you can see signs of progress.

IN THE LAST FEW WEEKS, HAVE YOU:

Felt fatigued?	Yes	No
Gained weight?	Yes	No
Felt unusually cold?	Yes	No
Been constipated?	Yes	No
Noticed hair loss?	Yes	No
Had skin problems?	Yes	No
Had nail problems?	Yes	No
Had an excessive appetite?	Yes	No
Had hearing problems?	Yes	No
Had voice problems?	Yes	No
Had difficulty swallowing?	Yes	No
Had a poor memory?	Yes	No
Had problems with concentration?	Yes	No
Felt anxious for no reason?	Yes	No
Felt depressed or low?	Yes	No

Add up the number of times you checked "Yes" and enter the number:

SCORING:
0-3 .... LOW
4-7 .... MODERATE
8-11 .... SIGNIFICANT
12+ .... EXTREME

What was your score? Don't forget to record it and retake the test after your first month and after your third month on the diet. Things may seem bleak now, but you're on the right path. We know that most thyroid disease today is caused by too much iodine. In the next chapter, I will explain in more detail why this happens and how the thyroid can fix itself, when given the chance.

Chapter Three

The #1 Cause of Thyroid Disease

The last chapter showed how essential good thyroid function is for life. It also explained that thyroid disease is what happens when thyroid cells either overgrow or make the wrong amount of hormones. So why does this happen? There are multiple factors at play. Some are the existential details of life; as important as these are, we cannot change them. Existential factors include gender, age, genetics, and economic status in one's society.

We know that thyroid disease becomes more common with age. Also, women get it five to eight times as often as men. A person is more likely to get thyroid disease if a parent or sibling has it. The more affluent a society is, the more likely its members get thyroid disease. It seems that children who experience fewer infections are more prone to autoimmune diseases later in life.

Other factors that govern thyroid disease relate to the environment in which we live, such as whether a person is subjected to radiation, or takes certain medications, or is exposed to toxicants. For instance, ionizing radiation directed toward the thyroid can be a culprit. In the past, doctors often used radiation to treat tonsillitis; today, it's only used for head and neck cancers. Several medications can also cause thyroid disease to start; the biggest culprits are those high in iodine, like amiodarone. Some toxic chemicals can raise the risk of thyroid disease, like BPA, mercury, or cadmium. However, toxic chemicals alone do not explain most thyroid disease; iodine is the main factor.

Consuming the wrong amount of iodine is the main driver of all types of thyroid disease, as well as much of thyroid growth abnormalities. Too little iodine, too much iodine, or fluctuations in iodine intake can all be culprits. We can measure iodine; we can control it; and now we know that we can use it to reverse thyroid disease.

HOW THYROID DISEASE HAPPENS

The thyroid needs iodine to make its hormones, but the two have a strained relationship. That is, the blood cannot carry that much iodine, so the thyroid needs to search for every speck of it in the blood and suck it in.

Iodine is dangerous stuff, and it is rarely found in nature. When iodine does occur in food, water, cosmetics, and nearly all other sources, it is in its less reactive form, called iodide. To make the thyroid hormones, the gland then turns the iodide into the more volatile version, iodine. The thyroid handles it like a scientist handles a strong acid, lining its cells with antioxidants like glutathione for protection. If the iodine spills, the thyroid cells become inflamed and cannot effectively make hormones. The immune system can then attack the inflamed cells, destroying them and compounding a person's lack of thyroid hormones. Nevertheless, it all starts with excess iodine.

We used to think that thyroid disease could not be cured. We now know that unless nearly all the cells are dead, the damage can be stopped, and the cells can be repaired if given a break from excessive iodine. We cannot get our iodine intake down to zero, nor would we need to. Nearly every food has some iodine. But you will see from the clinical trials that even a modest reduction in iodine intake is often enough to cure thyroid disease.

The Thyroid Reset Diet lowers a person's iodine intake enough to let the thyroid clear out the excess iodine that has slowed it down; the diet does so by removing the hidden sources of iodine in your food.

EXPLORING THE EVIDENCE

With thousands of studies published daily, it can be easy to find one or two studies that seem to support any pet theory. But scientists know to pay attention to the findings that show up repeatedly, from different types of research.

The three main types of research are:

1. Test tube studies
2. Epidemiologic studies that look at population trends
3. Interventional trials using some treatment of interest

In the case of iodine and thyroid disease, we have consensus from all three types of research.

From test tube studies, we know that too much iodine slows down the thyroid and causes the immune system to attack it. From epidemiologic studies, we know that populations that increase their iodine intake go on to develop more thyroid disease. Interventional trials have shown that people who are given more iodine get thyroid disease, while reducing people's iodine intake can often reverse thyroid disease.

Based on everything we know, it is fair to say that it is possible to reset thyroid disease with iodine regulation. It happens in the real world, and it is not just a random correlation. Since these ideas are so new, here is evidence from each of the three areas.

TEST TUBE STUDIES

Excess iodine can harm the thyroid either slowly or all at once; a single high dose can cause thyroid disease. This severe reaction is brought about by topical iodine, iodine supplements, and medications with iodine.[1,2]

The harm occurs because excess iodine directly slows down the thyroid, triggering the immune system to attack the thyroid. Scientists have watched how thyroid cells respond in test tubes when iodine is added; above a certain threshold, they slow down and become inflamed. When thyroid cells are taken from a person or an animal exposed to excessive iodine, they also see that the immune system is activated.

IODINE SLOWS THE THYROID

If you had a short-circuit in your home's wiring, the circuit breaker would be tripped and the lights would go out. Similarly, the circuit breaker is there to protect your home against surges of electricity. Your thyroid has a mechanism just like a circuit breaker to protect it against too much iodine. It is called the Wolff Chaikoff effect, and we have known about it since the 1950s.[3] Without this protective mechanism, excess iodine could lead to a fatal excess of thyroid hormones. We know the Wolff Chaikoff effect is real because it is the most effective way to stop a thyroid overload.

One of the most dangerous situations in thyroid disease is a hyperthyroid storm. This is a complication of Graves' hyperthyroidism, in which the thyroid levels are so high they can be lethal. The strongest way to stop the thyroid from producing all those hormones in this situation is a megadose of iodine—thanks to the Wolff Chaikoff effect.

The Wolff Chaikoff effect does not always shut down the thyroid, however. In some cases, the thyroid slows down for several weeks. A mild excess of iodine can then cause the thyroid to become somewhat slower than normal on an ongoing basis.

IODINE TRIGGERS THE IMMUNE SYSTEM

In addition to directly slowing the thyroid, excess iodine can cause the immune system to attack the gland. If this attack goes on long enough, the gland can become too damaged to work. But in most cases, the immune attack stops if the excess iodine is eliminated.

It turns out that there are three main steps to this process:

1. **FREE RADICAL FORMATION** Iodide is turned into the highly oxidative free radical iodine within the thyroid cells. In small amounts, it is good that iodine is volatile so that it binds to thyroglobulin and makes thyroid hormones. The thyroid cells make large amounts of antioxidants like glutathione to protect themselves from the free radicals of iodine. Healthy thyroglobulin may have as few as 13 iodine atoms stuck to it, but with excess iodine in the diet, this can be as many as 60 atoms.[4] The more iodine on thyroglobulin, the more likely the lymphocytes will attack it.[5]
2. **IMMUNE ALERT** As thyroid cells get inflamed, many of them die. This high rate of cell death sends an alert throughout the immune system. Lymphocytes are sent in from other parts of the body to find out what is going wrong inside the thyroid and get rid of it.[6,7]
3. **IMMUNE SYSTEM CONFUSION** When the lymphocytes target the inflammation coming from thyroid proteins, they begin to attack the thyroid cells by mistake.[8] Like collateral damage in times of war, the lymphocytes damage the thyroid machinery. They may also develop a taste for blood. The immune system becomes sensitized to the thyroid and can attack it more easily in the future.[9,10]

As bad as this all is, it can stop as soon as the excess iodine can be cleared out.

POPULATION STUDIES

Scientists observe large groups of people in all parts of the world. In particular, they have compared how much iodine people consume to how likely those same people are to develop thyroid disease.

In the past, getting too little iodine was a problem for much of the world's population. Many countries solved this problem by fortifying their salt with iodine. When they did so, that helped lower the rate of goiter among children. However, each country that fortified its salt with iodine has also seen increased thyroid disease.

In the largest review involving fifty studies, it was concluded that global iodine fortification has increased the risks of hypothyroidism and hyperthyroidism.[11]

Here are a few examples:

COUNTRY	YEAR OF IODINE FORTIFICATION	CHANGE IN THYROID DISEASE
Australia	1998	64 percent increase
Hungary	1998	950 percent increase
Poland	1997	300 percent increase
Zimbabwe	1995	300 percent increase

Source: Sun X, Shan Z, Teng W. Effects of Increased Iodine Intake on Thyroid Disorders. *Endocrinol Metab.* 2014;29(3):240–247. doi:10.3803/EnM.2014.29.3.240

FORTIFICATION IN THE UNITED STATES

Researchers from the Mayo Clinic in Minnesota tracked the rate of Hashimoto's thyroiditis in patients from 1935 to 1967. Within two years, the doctors saw an increase in autoimmune thyroid disease caused by iodine fortification.[12]

Starting with the first decade after iodine fortification, they documented a 4,800 percent increase in Hashimoto's disease. The earliest rates were 2.1 per every 100,000 persons; by the end of the study, it was up to 54.1 for women under 39 and 94.1 for those over 40.

FORTIFICATION IN DENMARK

Denmark is one of the most recent industrial nations to fortify its food with iodine. Denmark had a known rate for development of goiters, but its rates of hypothyroidism and hyperthyroidism were much lower than those of most industrialized countries. Because of the possible bad effects, they aimed to increase the population's intake of iodine by only 50 mcg per day. Thus, Denmark took a cautionary approach to dietary fortification. Any intentional modifications to vitamin or mineral intake were done only in conjunction with careful monitoring of pertinent health conditions.

The researchers monitored thyroid function in three ways, and they had begun the monitoring many years before iodization, so any trends could be clear. First, they chose a group of 4,649 people in two areas with differing levels of iodine intake. For each person, they carefully evaluated diet, health, and thyroid function. This group was later compared to a similar group of 3,570 people in 2005, well after iodine fortification had begun. Then they tracked the rate of diagnosis of hypo- or hyperthyroidism, as well as treatments for thyroid disease, including medications, surgery, and radio ablation. This was carried out among 550,000 people living in those same two areas. This was possible because of Denmark's central healthcare system.

In July 2000, the nation instituted a program that mandated the iodization of salt made for household use and for that used in commercial bread production. Yet just an extra 50 mcg of iodine led to increases in hypothyroidism, Hashimoto's thyroiditis, and Graves' disease, as well as thyroid surgery and prescriptions for thyroid medication. In the first three years alone, prescriptions for thyroid disease medications shot up by 42 percent. These changes did not just happen for a little while; they have continued for sixteen years now. Occurrences of autoimmune hypothyroidism went up by 53 percent, and Graves' disease went up by 50 percent.

The important point to take away from this is that the Danes were not overdosing on iodine. It was just that their iodine intake changed.

As much of a clear danger that excess iodine poses, major fluctuations of iodine can also be harmful, even if there is not an ongoing overdose. That is why regulating the amount of iodine you're getting daily from your foods and supplements is so crucial. The change in iodine intake also led to weight gain. Those with thyroid function on the low side of normal were found to weigh 8.8 pounds more than those with better thyroid levels.

The goal for Denmark's iodine fortification was a reduction in the incidence of goiter. But the study revealed that goiter and thyroid nodules were also largely influenced by smoking and alcohol use. In retrospect, the Danish study showed that reductions in alcohol and smoking could have lowered goiter by as much as was achieved with iodine fortification, without increasing the occurrence of thyroid disease.

Nearly every country that has fortified its food supply with iodine has seen the same results. Here are just three more examples: In 1995, Zimbabwe raised its iodine intake slightly and saw that hyperthyroidism went up 300 percent. Austria saw that occurrences of hyperthyroidism went up by as much as 64 percent after fortification began in 1998. Tasmania saw its rates similarly go up by over threefold; they also saw that remission from Graves' disease was highest when the iodine intakes were the lowest.[13]

The "Iodine Project"

Doctors of alternative medicine have a bias toward the use of vitamins and minerals. They assume that these supplements are always safer because they are natural. In the early 2000s, a gynecologist launched an iodine frenzy that continues to this day. He was inspired by studies showing that iodine could help reduce the pain of fibrocystic breast disease.

His ideas were so intriguing that I reached out and asked to speak to him personally. He was a gracious man and gave freely of his time. After our first call, he shipped me a large box as a gift. In it was every word he had ever written on iodine and all the references. I read all of it, at first with a sense of excitement about the new finding. Then I became concerned when I noticed that most of the references were not to external sources; they were to his own work. I started to have doubts, and I read the independently published data on iodine. It all made me uncomfortable. He was a kind person who meant well, but the unavoidable conclusion was that he was wrong.

Most of the studies on fibrocystic breast disease involved a pretty high dose of iodine, usually 5,000 mcg.[14] This doctor reasoned that if a high dose of iodine helped these women, then they must have been nutritionally lacking iodine. He argued that the conventional wisdom about people needing only a few hundred mcg must be wrong because these women seemed to benefit from much more.

Nutrients are chemicals with complex properties. In small amounts, they can be essential parts of normal reactions. In larger amounts, however, they can have drug-like effects that have nothing to do with fulfilling their role as nutrients. If I cut my hand and it got infected, I might use 10,000 mcg of iodine to kill the bacteria. But that doesn't mean I'm iodine deficient, or that my body needs that much iodine to function. For example, a megadose of niacin can lower cholesterol; that does not mean that everyone with high cholesterol is niacin deficient.

Along with being wrong, this approach can be harmful. Numerous cases have been reported in which people developed thyroid disease from following this regimen.[15,16] Most tragic are the stories of this doctor's followers giving recommendations to pregnant women and thereby causing major birth defects.[17]

***

Because of these misconceptions about iodine, stories like Julia's, below, are common:

Case Story: Julia

Julia came to see Dr. Khoshaba to get her thyroid function back to normal. Julia had a baby nineteen months prior to the visit, and she mentioned that new symptoms had been developing during the last year. Her symptoms included weight loss, a racing heart, an enlarged neck, and hair loss. Since Integrative Health doctors focus on thyroid disease, we do thyroid blood tests on all patients before their first visit, to save time. Julia's tests showed that her thyroid was making way too much hormone. She had serious hyperthyroidism, but she did not have signs of Graves' disease, its most common cause.

Julia told Dr. Khoshaba that she had been taking iodine drops for a little over a year, on the advice of a functional medicine doctor. She was told to take 30 drops per day. Dr. Khoshaba found that each drop had 150 mcg of iodine. Julia had some reservations, and did not always take the full amount, but she rarely took less than 20 drops per day. Dr. Khoshaba ran the math and told Julia she was getting between 3,000 and 4,500 mcg of extra iodine each day, and that some people could get thyroid disease from just a few hundred extra micrograms.

Dr. Khoshaba had her stop the iodine and gave her treatments to slow her thyroid and lower the side effects. Within six weeks, Julia was feeling better. Within seven months, Julia was feeling fine and had normal thyroid function, without any medication.

INTERVENTIONAL TRIALS

So far, results of test-tube studies and population trends have been discussed. All pieces of evidence are important, but the most important data come from seeing what happens to people in real time. Human studies consistently show two things: First, if you give people extra iodine, many of them develop thyroid disease. Second, if people with thyroid disease reduce their iodine intake, the disease often goes away.

IODINE SUPPLEMENTATIONS CAUSE THYROID DISEASE

A recent study showed that iodine supplementation slows thyroid function. The higher the dose, the worse the effect, but even the smallest doses were harmful. In the study, 256 healthy adults, free of thyroid disease, were given a dose of supplemental iodine or a placebo. The iodine doses ranged from as little as 100 mcg to as high as 2,000 mcg. Most multivitamins that contain iodine are labeled to contain 100 to 175 mcg of iodine. No changes were seen in the placebo group, but many of those taking 100 mcg of iodine saw thyroid disease emerge within four weeks. Of those at the 2,000 mcg intake level, 31 percent developed thyroid disease.[18]

In another study to evaluate the tolerability of iodine supplementation, a group of adults were given 200 mcg of iodine or a placebo for twelve months. Over 10 percent of those given iodine developed thyroid disease, but that did not happen to those on the placebo. When the iodine was discontinued, the thyroid function normalized.[19]

REVERSING THYROID DISEASE

Here is where it gets exciting. It's been proven that it *is* possible to reverse thyroid disease.

In a dramatic human study, people with hypothyroidism caused by Hashimoto's were assigned to a low-iodine diet or to eat as they normally do. Of those on the low-iodine diet, 78.3 percent were cured of the Hashimoto's within three months.

These patients were significantly hypothyroid. Normal TSH scores were defined in this study as 0.41 to 4.43 IU/mL. As noted earlier, a high TSH score means the thyroid is sluggish; a low one means it is overactive. These patients' TSH scores started as a group average of 14.28. The levels are not subtle; they reflect severe hypothyroidism.

Within three months of regulating only their iodine intake, nearly all their scores were normal. The group average came down from over 14 to 3.18! Of those whose scores did not return to normal, nevertheless there were still improvements, typically by 50 percent or more. For example, one such patient started with a TSH score of 200, which was reduced to 100. That's still far from ideal, but it is making rapid progress. The study's control group had no such reversal of thyroid disease.

Some of the study's participants did not get any benefits; however, their urinary iodine levels had been much higher than of those who did get better. In short, they were still getting a lot of iodine. There are two possibilities for this: either they did not try as hard to follow the guidelines, or they had inadvertent sources of dietary iodine that they were not aware of. We use the same approach in the Thyroid Reset Diet. That is, if someone does not seem to respond, we test again to see if the person got the iodine to a low enough level.

One of several fascinating points from this study was that the baseline iodine intake was not different between the responders and the non-responders. That is, iodine regulation helped those who had average intakes of iodine just as much as it helped those with high intake. This is one of the reasons I do not ask people to test their iodine before starting the Thyroid Reset Diet. If someone does not respond, iodine tests can then be helpful to make sure there was no hidden source of iodine that was holding back improvement.

Another group of researchers checked to see if similar results could be obtained in those who were hypothyroid but did not have clear signs of Hashimoto's. They chose a group of patients with a median age of 52, all with hypothyroidism. The patients were told to avoid all medications and supplements containing iodine, as well as sea vegetables and any other high-iodine foods. The researchers gave the participants no treatments or recommendations, and none of them were prescribed thyroid medication. Within just eight weeks, 63.6 percent of these participants returned to normal thyroid function. As in the prior study, those who did get completely better still improved somewhat. Also, ultrasound findings showed improvement in many of the patients after iodine reduction.[20]

In conclusion, you can see how the tiniest changes in iodine intake can have a tremendous effect on your thyroid function. Now let's delve into those sources of excess iodine.

Chapter Four

Invisible Iodine

You know that too much iodine can be dangerous to your thyroid and that a reduction in iodine can reverse thyroid disease. Now is the time to look at the major sources of excess iodine in our diets.

First, let us make sense of the exact amounts of iodine that are best. Here, let's look at where you should fall on the spectrum toward reversing thyroid disease, and where you should be in terms of maintenance. Then I'll discuss some of the biggest hidden sources of iodine and how you can work around them.

THE IODINE INDEX

Much of what we know about how different levels of iodine affect our health comes from the World Health Organization (WHO). Its researchers have compared thyroid disease and iodine intake in every country in the world. They have paid close attention to changes that occur after a country starts adding iodine to its food. As a result, the

WHO has compiled this information and formed guidelines to help reduce the risks of thyroid disease through safer use of iodine.

As part of WHO guidelines, there is a six-level spectrum of iodine intake. Because there is no easy way to track a person's iodine intake, the Thyroid Reset Diet organizes foods into a simple Green Light, Yellow Light, and Red Light model. This model fits the WHO guidelines and helps you keep track of your iodine levels. Further, Chapter Seven has complete food lists organized by Green Light, Yellow Light, and Red Light categories.

Here is a summary table to give you the overall idea:

IODINE INDEX: SUMMARY

	WHO LEVEL	TYPES OF ILLNESS	DIETARY IODINE INTAKE
	1	Endemic goiter Congenital hypothyroidism	< 20 mcg
	2	Pediatric goiter, low rate of adult disease	20–49 mcg
Green Light (Reset or Maintenance Phase)	3	Lowest disease rate + reversal of autoimmune thyroid disease, hypothyroidism	50–99 mcg
Yellow Light (Maintenance Phase)	4	Low disease rate	100–199 mcg
Red Light	5	Iodine-induced hyperthyroidism, autoimmune thyroid disease, goiter, hypothyroidism	200–299 mcg
	6	Hypothyroidism, goiter, autoimmune thyroid disease	> 300 mcg

Sources: WHO. Urinary Iodine Concentrations for Determining Iodine Status in Populations. World Health Organization. 2013; Chung JH. Low Iodine Diet for Preparation for Radioactive Iodine Therapy in Differentiated Thyroid Carcinoma in Korea. *J Clin Endocrinol Metab.* 2013;28(3):157–163. doi:10.3803/EnM.2013.28.3.157; Park JT, Hennessey JV. Two-Week Low Iodine Diet Is Necessary for Adequate Outpatient Preparation for Radioiodine rhTSH Scanning in Patients Taking Levothyroxine. *Thyroid.* 2004;14(1):57–63. doi:10.1089/105072504322783858; Luster M, Clarke SE, Dietlein M, et al. Guidelines for Radioiodine Therapy of Differentiated Thyroid Cancer. *Eur J Nucl Med Mol Imaging.* 2008;35(10):1941–1959. doi:10.1007/s00259-008-0883-1; Henjum S, Brantsæter AL, Kurniasari A, et al. Suboptimal Iodine Status and Low Iodine Knowledge in Young Norwegian Women. *Nutrients.* 2018;10(7):941. doi:10.3390/nu10070941; Delange F. Iodine Requirements During Pregnancy, Lactation, and the Neonatal Period and Indicators of Optimal Iodine Nutrition. *Public Health Nutr.* 2007;10(12):1571–1580. doi:10.1017/S1368980007360941

LEVEL 1: HIGHEST RATES OF GOITER

People consuming under 20 mcg of iodine a day are suffering a severe iodine deficiency. Thyroid disease is common here, mainly goiter, which may affect as many as 30 percent of children. Intake this low used to be found only in regions with iodine-deficient soil, limited food options, and no iodine-fortified salt. Today, it is nonexistent.

In 1990, 112 countries were at this level. In 1991, the U.N. World Summit for Children set out to change this. By 2014, the number of severely iodine-deficient nations was zero. The trend away from severe iodine deficiency is a huge win for the world. However, it has correlated with more countries moving into unsafe levels of iodine, which is not good.

LEVEL 2: MORE GOITER, LESS AUTOIMMUNE THYROID DISEASE

This is a moderate iodine deficiency. People at this level consume 20 to 49 mcg per day. The rates of goiter are higher than normal at level 2, but Hashimoto's disease and hypothyroidism are rare. Regions in level 2 do not have iodine fortification, but they do have more diverse diets than those that used to be in level 1. In 2014, only seven countries were at this level: Algeria, Angola, Central African Republic, Ethiopia, Gambia, Haiti, and Vanuatu.[1]

LEVEL 3: BEST TO REVERSE THYROID DISEASE

This is also the Reset phase of the Thyroid Reset Diet. Eating only Green Light foods will keep you in level 3. You will ingest roughly 50 to 99 mcg of iodine per day. Pediatric goiter is slightly higher than the baseline, but adult thyroid disease is at its lowest at this level. This is true for adult autoimmune thyroid disease, hypothyroidism, and subclinical hypothyroidism. This level can also be used therapeutically to reverse thyroid disease. Diets at this level include a wide range of unprocessed foods and avoid iodine-fortified salt and sources of excess iodine.

LEVEL 4: SAFE FOR THOSE WITHOUT THYROID DISEASE

The Maintenance phase of the Thyroid Reset Diet extends from the bottom of level 3 to the top of level 4. To stay in level 4, you can have unlimited amounts of foods from the Green Light list and up to two servings of foods from the Yellow Light list. This is considered general iodine sufficiency, or 100 to 199 mcg per day. This is the level at which most types of thyroid disease are at their lowest in children and are still low in adults. This level is often not low enough to reverse the symptoms that came from iodine excess and may not keep patients with thyroid disease stable. Pregnant and breastfeeding women may be below their optimal iodine. Typical diets at this level include iodine-fortified salt and some processed foods.

LEVEL 5: ABOVE ADEQUATE

Here, 200 to 299 mcg of iodine per day is considered above sufficiency. This is the point at which disease from excess iodine starts to show up. Frequent use of Yellow Light foods or occasional use of Red Light foods can put you into this range. This group continues to grow. We now have fifty-two countries in this range, including the United States.

High levels of iodine can cause some of the same symptoms as iodine deficiency, including goiter. They also cause iodine-induced hyperthyroidism, Hashimoto's thyroiditis, and Graves' disease. Most modern diets with iodine-fortified salt and that are high in processed foods fall in this range. The World Health Organization categorized levels 5 and 6 as being at increased risk of iodine-induced thyroid disease. The United States and Central and South America are among the regions at risk.[2]

When we take a more detailed look at the U.S. population, we see that average figures can be deceiving. I once heard a professor say that a person with his head in an oven and his feet in a bucket of ice might have an average temperature that was exactly right. Our situation is somewhat similar. The average intake is above ideal, but some people consume way too much iodine and some may get too little.

For example, pregnant women need more iodine than nonpregnant adults, but nearly 7 percent of them may be getting too little.[3] The ideal range in this case is 150 to 250 mcg per day. Note that this range for pregnant women is higher and narrower than for those in the non-pregnant state. Yet it is still possible to get too much iodine during pregnancy, a situation that can be a problem for those who have existing thyroid disease or a susceptibility to it. At the same time, many subgroups get too much iodine. When we look at various ages and ethnicities of Americans, we see that large numbers of people are overconsuming iodine.

PERCENTAGE OF THE U.S. POPULATION AT UNSAFE IODINE LEVEL (≥ 200 mcg/L)

GENDER	ETHNICITY	AGE				
		20–29	30–39	40–49	50–59	60–69
Female	NHW	36%	35%	31%	33%	34%
	NHB	19%	23%	33%	37%	33%
	MA	33%	41%	32%	40%	35%
Male	NHW	37%	35%	46%	41%	48%
	NHB	29%	27%	33%	32%	44%
	MA	35%	47%	45%	40%	47%

NHW = non-Hispanic white
NHB = non-Hispanic black
MA = Mexican-American

Sources: Caldwell KL, Makhmudov A, Ely E, Jones RL, Wang RY. Iodine Status of the U.S. Population, National Health and Nutrition Examination Survey, 2005–2006 and 2007–2008. *Thyroid.* 2011;21(4):1–9. doi:10.1089/thy.2010.0077; (no title) https://www.ign.org/cm_data/2011_Caldwell_Iodine_status_of_the_US_population_NHNES_2005_06_and_07_08_Thyroid.pdf. Accessed May 14, 2020

LEVEL 6: EXCESSIVE

This level presents an overt iodine danger, in that people are consuming over 299 mcg of iodine per day. All types of thyroid disease become more prevalent in children, adults, and pregnant women. These populations have iodine-fortified salt and high intakes of iodine from processed foods and supplements. Frequent consumption of Red Light foods brings people up to this level. As bad as this is, there are now five countries in this range, and the list is growing.

INVISIBLE SOURCES OF IODINE

There are eight main sources of iodine that can provide amounts harmful to your thyroid. Some of these sources always contain too much iodine, while others have amounts that fluctuate greatly. The sources of invisible iodine include the following:

Food

- Baked goods
- Dairy products
- Eggs
- Salt
- Seafood and sea vegetables

Other Sources

- Cosmetics
- Vaginal douches
- Medications
- Dietary supplements

Let us look at each category and see how they could all fit together to create a state of iodine excess.

BAKED GOODS

Grains in themselves contain no significant amounts of iodine. This is true for grains both with and without gluten. It is also true for flour, as well as for cracked and rolled-grain products. Examples include white and whole wheat flour, old-fashioned rolled oats, and bulgur wheat.

Yet commercially baked goods commonly contain unsafe levels of iodine, and the content has been getting higher in recent decades.

FOOD	MAXIMUM IODINE PER SERVING
Bread, white, enriched	610 mcg
Bread, whole wheat	530 mcg
Bread, multigrain	440 mcg
Bagel, plain, toasted	410 mcg

Sources: U.S. Food and Drug Administration. *Total Diet Study: Elements Results Summary Statistics—Market Baskets 2006 through 2013*. USDA, 2014; Mason R. Chlorella and Spirulina: Green Supplements for Balancing the Body. *Altern Complement Ther*. June. 2001;28(2020):161-165; National Institutes of Health. Iodine: Fact Sheet for Health Professionals.NIH. Iodine—Health Professional Fact Sheet. *Natl Institutes Heal*. 2011:1-6. https://ods.od.nih.gov/factsheets/Iodine-HealthProfessional/. Accessed August 14, 2020

Why do commercially baked goods have such high levels of iodine? When asked, most dieticians attribute the source of the iodine to iodized dough conditioners. Some have claimed that these conditioners are no longer used in modern bread production.

Yet the facts are not consistent. When researchers analyze baked products, they often still find unsafe levels of iodine. In a study described in the *Journal of Clinical Endocrinology and Metabolism*, researchers found that commercial bread could have as much as 1,174 mcg of iodine per slice. Some bread products list the iodized dough conditioners in their ingredient list, but most do not—and some of these are the breads with those unsafe levels of iodine.[4]

It seems that either some bakeries may not disclose their use of iodized dough conditioners or there may be other sources of iodine that have not been disclosed. In short, it appears that there is no way to know how much iodine you might get when you purchase commercially baked goods.

The best course of action to protect your thyroid, therefore, is to avoid all commercially baked products. Grains and other flour products do not, in themselves, contain significant amounts of iodine, so those goods that are baked at home will be low in iodine and safe to eat.

DAIRY PRODUCTS

Of all the various food categories, dairy products may be the largest contributors of iodine.[5] They may also be the most variable sources.

For example, the amount of iodine in milk products can vary by more than a factor of 10, from batch to batch.

FOOD	MAXIMUM IODINE PER SERVING
Milk, skim	360mcg
Yogurt, low-fat, fruit-flavored	228 mcg
Milk, low-fat (2%)	150 mcg
Milkshake, chocolate, fast-food	126 mcg
Milk, whole	122 mcg
Yogurt, whole milk, unsweetened	30 mcg
Cream cheese	30 mcg

Sources: U.S. Food and Drug Administration. *Total Diet Study: Elements Results Summary Statistics—Market Baskets 2006 through 2013.* USDA, 2014; Mason R. Chlorella and Spirulina: Green Supplements for Balancing the Body. *Altern Complement Ther.* June. 2001;28(2020):161-165; National Institutes of Health. Iodine: Fact Sheet for Health Professionals. NIH. Iodine—Health Professional Fact Sheet. *Natl institutes Heal.* 2011:1-6. https://ods.od.nih.gov/factsheets/Iodine-HealthProfessional/. Accessed August 14, 2020

Why is milk high in iodine? The main reason is that farmers use iodine to sanitize the cows' teats. This practice has gone on for over a century, but with the rise of resistant bacteria, the use of iodine as a dairy sanitizer is greater now than it was as recently as the 1990s. Iodine is also an irritant to the udders and a significant expense to the farmers, so its use is questionable even from an economic standpoint. Indeed, non-iodine teat sanitizers have become commercially available as of 2019 and may soon become more widely used.

Also, cows are often given supplemental iodine in the minerals used to fortify their feed. They may also be given fishmeal, which is high in iodine,[6,7] as a low-cost protein source.

We have assumed that the increased rates of thyroid disease in America was because of iodine in salt. Interestingly, the UK saw an identical increase in thyroid disease over the same time period, yet they did not fortify their salt. However, starting in the 1930s, both the United States and the UK began using iodine to fortify dairy feed cattle.[8]

Studies have found an average of 427 mcg per liter of iodine in conventional milk versus 241 mcg per liter in organic.[9] So, although organic dairy products may be lower in iodine, their numbers are still too high to be used freely by those with thyroid disease. The reason organic milk is thought to be lower in iodine is that cows fed organic feed consume higher amounts of naturally occurring iodine-binding glucosinolates from rapeseed and glycosides from clover.[10]

Are there safer dairy foods? Yes, non-dairy products like soy milk, coconut yogurt, vegan yogurt, and hemp cheese are readily available. In the past, many of these products had iodine from the seaweed extracts used in them; nowadays, nearly none of them do.

All dairy foods have some iodine, but the amounts are lower in hard cheeses and sour cream. In the Maintenance phase, these lower-iodine dairy products can be used if the amounts and frequencies are considered.

It's clear that baked goods and dairy products have high amounts of iodine, but it was not always that way. Since 1982, the FDA's *Total Diet Study* (TDS) has measured iodine concentrations in certain foods in four different regions of America. They found that when the years 1982–1991 and 2003–2011 are compared, the amount of iodine in twenty-three of the top twenty-five dietary sources of iodine all increased, some by as much as 300 percent.[11] Baked goods and dairy foods are among those most directly influencing these statistics. The increasingly unsafe amounts of iodine in the foods are thought to be one of the reasons occurrence of thyroid disease has risen over this same time period.

Here are a few more examples of foods that have shown increased levels of iodine compared to prior years. Bear in mind that a healthy intake of iodine is just under 200 mcg per day.

ELEVATED IODINE LEVELS, 2006–2013

FOOD	IODINE CONTENT IN SERVING (MCG PER 100 G)
Sherbet, fruit-flavored	1,480 mcg
Cake, white, with icing	1,300 mcg
Sugar cookie	750 mcg
Candy, hard, any flavor	680 mcg
Commercial bread, white	610 mcg

FOOD	IODINE CONTENT IN SERVING (MCG PER 100 G)
Commercial bread, whole wheat	530 mcg
Meal replacement, ready-to-drink, any flavor	490 mcg
Commercial bagel, plain, toasted	410 mcg
Donut, cake type, from donut store	350 mcg
Popsicle, fruit-flavored	290 mcg
Eggs, boiled	230 mcg
Breakfast tart/toaster pastry	170 mcg
Swiss cheese	150 mcg
Pizza cheese and pepperoni, carry-out	140 mcg
Cantaloupe, frozen	130 mcg
Milkshake, chocolate, fast-food	100 mcg
Beef stir-fry with vegetables, Chinese carry-out	98 mcg
Ice cream, regular, vanilla	95 mcg
Fishsticks, baked	91 mcg
Candy bar, milk chocolate	87 mcg
Prune juice	61 mcg
Fruit cocktail, canned in light syrup	54 mcg
Decaffeinated coffee, flavored	53 mcg

Source: U.S. Food and Drug Administration. *Total Diet Study: Elements Results Summary Statistics—Market Baskets 2006 through 2013.*. USDA, 2014

EGGS

With regard to eggs, the iodine is solely found in the yolks. Based on limited data, organic eggs do not seem to have different amounts of iodine compared to conventionally produced eggs.[12]

FOOD	MAX IODINE PER SERVING
Eggs scrambled with oil	250 mcg
Eggs, boiled	230 mcg

Source: U.S. Food and Drug Administration. *Total Diet Study: Elements Results Summary Statistics—Market Baskets 2006 through 2013.*MD: USDA, 2014.; Mason R. Chlorella and Spirulina: Green Supplements for Balancing the Body. *Altern Complement Ther.* June. 2001;28(2020):161-165; National Institutes of Health. Iodine: Fact Sheet for Health Professionals. NIH. Iodine—Health Professional Fact Sheet. *Natl institutes Heal.* 2011:1–6. https://ods.od.nih.gov/factsheets/Iodine-HealthProfessional/. Accessed August 14, 2020

Therefore, egg whites can be freely used without restriction during any phase of the Thyroid Reset Diet. If you avoid eggs owing to other dietary guidelines or long-standing allergies, however, continue to do so.

SEAFOOD AND SEA VEGETABLES

Seawater contains substantial amounts of iodine, and iodine is a source of free radicals. Therefore, all life in the oceans must be adapted to deal with more iodine than does land-based life. Many types of seafood have concentrated iodine to significant degrees, and all types of sea vegetables do as well.

Here are some examples of seafood with unsafe amounts of iodine:

FOOD	MAX IODINE PER SERVING
Cod, Pacific	315 mcg
Pollock	280 mcg
Haddock	227 mcg
Lobster, prepared	185 mcg
Oyster, prepared	109 mcg
Anglerfish	100 mcg
Abalone	97 mcg
Clams, canned	66 mcg

Sources: U.S. Food and Drug Administration. *Total Diet Study: Elements Results Summary Statistics - Market Baskets 2006 through 2013*. USDA, 2014; Mason R. Chlorella and Spirulina: Green Supplements for Balancing the Body. *Altern Complement Ther*. June. 2001;28(2020):161-165; National Institutes of Health. Iodine: Fact Sheet for Health Professionals. NIH. August 14, 2020

Since seafood intake can provide health benefits,[13] I worked hard to find types that had consistently safe levels of iodine and include them in the diet, rather than exclude all seafood. Some of the safe options are scallops, squid, rainbow or river trout, and walleye tuna. Although seafood and sea vegetables both are high sources of iodine, the levels in seafood are more predictable.

The single food category with the highest amount of iodine by far is sea vegetables. Indeed, these are in a class by themselves. A single serving of many kinds of sea vegetables can contain hundreds of times more than the safe upper limit for iodine.

FOOD	IODINE PER SERVING
Kelp, granules	81,650 mcg
Kelp, powdered	23,530 mcg
Kelp, whole	19,970 mcg
Wild kelp, capsules	13,560 mcg
Kombu	13,500 mcg
Sea palm	8,710 mcg
Knotted wrack	6,460 mcg
Hijiki	6,290 mcg
Wakame	4,310 mcg
Bladderwrack	2,760 mcg
Dulse	720 mcg

Sources: U.S. Food and Drug Administration. *Total Diet Study: Elements Results Summary Statistics—Market Baskets 2006 through 2013.* USDA, 2014; Mason R. Chlorella and Spirulina: Green Supplements for Balancing the Body. *Altern Complement Ther.* June. 2001;28(2020):161–165; National Institutes of Health. Iodine: Fact Sheet for Health Professionals. NIH. Iodine—Health Professional Fact Sheet. *Natl institutes Heal.* 2011:1–6. https://ods.od.nih.gov/factsheets/Iodine-HealthProfessional/. Accessed August 14, 2020

The Thyroid Reset Diet's Maintenance phase does allow for chlorella and spirulina, but is it bad to otherwise avoid sea vegetables? They do have essential nutrients, beneficial fibers, and polyphenols. However, when you consider the risks involved, it seems clear that those prone to thyroid disease would do well to avoid these foods.

Both hypo- and hyperthyroidism are more common in populations with higher intakes of sea vegetables.[14,15,16] Sea vegetables from all parts of the world are also known to carry unsafe amounts of arsenic, cadmium, lead, and mercury.[17] Studies have also shown that increased consumption of sea vegetables can correlate with a 3.8 times risk increase for thyroid cancer in menopausal women.[18] Additionally, some health agencies advocate for restrictions on seafood intake in pregnant and lactating women, owing to the unsafe amounts of iodine and heavy metals.[19]

Case Story: Deidre

Deidre was the chair of a volunteer organization that helped disadvantaged women. She saw one of my doctors because she suspected thyroid disease. Her primary-care physician had already screened her and said she was fine.

But Deidre still had doubts because she was too tired to keep up with her normal activities. When she was tested, she was found to have high levels of thyroid antibodies and thyroid hormone levels that were on the edge of normal and well outside of optimal. When asked about her diet, she mentioned that she and her family ate seaweed snacks most days.

After avoiding these iodine-containing supplements and other high-iodine foods, she started feeling better within a few weeks. On her next retest, her thyroid levels were nearly optimal and her antibodies were negative.

SALT

One of the biggest determinants of success in reducing iodine consumption is how well you define your salt sources. Actually, this is one of the easiest food swaps to make. You do not have to limit your salt intake, you just need to use salt that does not have high amounts of iodine.

Commercial salts can have iodine added in or the iodine can be naturally occurring. It turns out that iodized salt is not the only salt you should avoid; popular forms of salt like sea salt or Himalayan salt may also have significant amounts of iodine. Sea salt is completely variable in its iodine content. One assay showed that sea salt could contain from 0 to 114 mcg per teaspoon, even though all the samples came from a small geographic area.[20]

Unlike other types of salt, sea salt does contain minerals besides sodium and chloride. But magnesium is the only mineral that occurs in amounts high enough to be useful. Celtic is one brand of sea salt that has some low-iodine options. Their products Flower of the

Ocean, or fleur de sel, has light gray coarse and light gray fine grains that are safe for regular use. If you are a fan of sea salt, use these; otherwise, stick with iodine-free salt. Note that other products by this same company do not have safe levels of iodine.

IODINE-FREE SALT	SALT WITH IODINE
Celtic light gray sea salt	Celtic brand makai salt
Maldon sea salt	Pink Himalayan salt
Diamond kosher salt	Table salt—iodized
Morton's kosher salt	Sea salt—non-iodized
Table salt—non-iodized	Sea salt—iodized
Pickling/canning salt	Real Salt
Canning salt	Lite-Salt
Nu-Salt	

Surprisingly, Himalayan salt appears to be higher in iodine than regular iodized salt, so it is not a good option for those with thyroid disease. According to one test, its iodine levels may be "around 0.1g/kg."[21] To convert the information to useful units, consider that this would be equal to 100 mcg of iodine per gram of salt. Iodized table salt in the United States has 45 mcg of iodine added to every gram of salt.[22] So, if you were to switch to Himalayan salt, while avoiding processed foods, you might raise your iodine intake from as little as 30 mcg (30 percent of 2 grams × 54 mcg/g) to as much as 400 mcg (100 mcg/g × 4 grams). Luckily, when it comes to salt, you have plenty of good options, like kosher salt or the Celtic gray sea salt.

OTHER SOURCES OF INVISIBLE IODINE

As important as food is, it is not the only source of invisible iodine. Cosmetics, medications, and supplements can contain massive amounts of iodine. For anyone exposed to or obtaining iodine from these sources, know that these may be main drivers of thyroid disease.

COSMETICS

One of the most shocking things I learned was that personal-care products could be invisible sources of iodine. Many forms of iodine are used in these personal-care products, which range from mascara and eyeliner, to shampoos, hair conditioners, and hair sprays, to skin lotions and sunscreens. Could they have enough iodine to matter? Let's run some numbers.

Several ingredients in personal-care products contain iodine, but the most common one is polyvinylpyrrolidone, or PVP. PVP is 12 percent iodine by weight.[23] The amounts vary by product, but facial moisturizers may have 1 to 5 percent PVP,[24] and conditioners are often at 0.5 to 3 percent.[25]

Human studies have shown that long-term exposure to topical iodine products can cause thyroid disease.[26] The use of iodine as a skin antiseptic after a cesarean section has been shown to disrupt thyroid function in mothers.[27] Infants have been shown to develop thyroid abnormalities when iodine is used as a skin antiseptic before delivery.[28]

In medical centers where the staff was using iodine-based hand products, 39 percent of the staff was found to have unsafe iodine levels.[29] Because of this, the FDA recently banned all iodine-containing antiseptics from hand sanitizers and antiseptic soaps.[30] So far, the use of iodine in cosmetics has not been addressed.

Iodine is not absorbed instantly, and it won't be absorbed if it is placed on a tiny area of skin. However, topical iodine can be absorbed on the skin in as little as 2 minutes and with as little as 2 cubic centimeters of exposed skin[31]—this is about the size of a dime. Not all of it is absorbed, but enough is that it does matter. Studies vary, but no less than 4.5 percent of iodine is likely absorbed when applied to healthy, intact skin.[32,33]

Take facial moisturizers as an example. A common application of a moisturizer can contain 15 grams (15,000,000 mcg). At even 3 percent PVP, this equals 450,000 mcg of PVP. With PVP containing 12 percent iodine, there is now 54,000 mcg of iodine. With 4.5 percent absorption, there could still be up to 2,430 mcg of iodine absorbed. Of course, there are many scenarios in which these numbers could be higher, but this shows that the amounts can be significant.

The main ingredients to watch out for include:

- Ammonium iodide
- Potassium iodide
- Sodium iodide
- Iodoform
- PVP-iodine
- Hydroxypropyl bistrimonium diiodide
- TEA-hydroiodide
- Ethiodized oil
- Iodopropynyl butylcarbamate
- Seaweed extracts: *Fucus vesiculosus* extract, *Laminaria digitata* extract, kelp extract

How common are these ingredients? I searched a shopping site for the top ten products in the categories of night creams and conditioners. For night creams, four out of ten had at least one of these listed ingredients. For conditioners, it was three of ten. Products that were marketed as being "natural" were just as likely to have iodine, but when they did, it was more commonly from one of the seaweed extracts.

Some products are not likely relevant because they are used in such tiny amounts or they may not come into contact with much skin surface. Examples of these include hair sprays, mascara, and eyeliner. So, overall, the products worth checking for iodine content include:

- Shampoos
- Conditioners
- Sunscreen
- Skin moisturizer
- Facial moisturizer

It is worth taking the time to be sure you are not exposing yourself to unintentional iodine through your skincare products. Take a few minutes and compare this list of ingredients with the ingredients in your products. If your product contains iodine, look for options that do not. Thankfully, it is easy to find cosmetics and skincare products that are free of iodine.

VAGINAL DOUCHES

In another example of personal-care products, many vaginal douche formulations contain iodine. Studies have shown that usage of an iodine-containing vaginal douche can cause exposure to iodine levels that could be unsafe for the woman and would be unsafe for a fetus if the woman is pregnant.[34]

Here are the action steps for cosmetics:

1. Read the labels on all your beauty products. If products do not have a full ingredient list, check online or request them from the manufacturer.
2. Avoid all products that use iodine-containing ingredients.
3. You can also find a list of approved cosmetic brands on your resource page www.thyroidresetdiet.com/resources.

Case Story: Elaine

Elaine was taking desiccated thyroid for hypothyroidism, but she was still not feeling well. She had lost nearly half her hair before finally being diagnosed with thyroid disease. She tried several different forms of thyroid medication and countless "hair vitamins," but her hair kept falling out. Finally, when she went on natural thyroid, it stopped falling out but it did not grow back. She and her doctor were never able to get her hormone levels adjusted satisfactorily. When she raised the dose, her scores would go too high; when she lowered it, they went too low.

When a doctor at Integrative Health reviewed Elaine's possible iodine sources, her biggest culprit was found to be her skin cream. Based on the ingredient list, she was getting as much as 2,300 mcg per day from it!

After ten weeks on the Thyroid Reset Diet, her thyroid levels steadied. She was able to use less medicine and bring her thyroid levels back to normal. Within six weeks, her hair loss stopped. By three months, she was happy to see tiny new hairs growing in!

MEDICATIONS

Medications containing iodine can be one of the more common triggers for thyroid disease. In one study, 11 percent of the patients consulting for thyroid disorders had been exposed to excessive iodine from drugs.[35]

Following is a list of medications that have hidden sources of iodine. If your doctor has prescribed one of these for you, do not stop taking it without speaking to him or her. But let your doctor know that you wish to regulate your iodine in hopes of improving your thyroid function, and see if there is an iodine-free option for you.

Most medications that can trigger thyroid disease are those not chosen lightly. They are often used in situations where, even though they may cause thyroid disease, the conditions being treated are even more urgent. One of the few instances where iodine exposure from medications can often be avoided is when the iodine is used as a contrast agent. In most of these cases, gadolinium can be substituted for iodine; versions of its use since 2010 are well tolerated and generally are good alternatives to iodine.[36]

Here is a list of most medications that can be sources of iodine:

Oral Medication

- Amiodarone
- Benziodarone

- Calcium iodide
- Diiodohydroxyquin (Yodoxin)
- R-Gen
- Echothiophate iodide ophthalmic solution (phosphine)
- Hydriodic acid syrup
- Iodochlorhydroxyquin (Entro-Vioform)
- Iodinated glycerol (Iophen)
- Idoxuridine ophthalmic solution (Herplex)
- Isopropamide iodide (Darbid)
- (KI) Potassium iodine
- Mudrane
- Lugol's Solution
- Niacinamide hydroiodide
- Ponaris nasal emollient
- Supersaturated potassium iodide (SSKI)

Injectable Solutions

- Sodium iodide

Topical Antiseptics

- Diiodohydroxyquin cream (Vytone)
- Iodine tincture
- Iodochlorhydroxyquin cream (Vioform)
- Cellasene
- Iodoform gauze (NuGauze)
- Povidone-iodine (Betadine)

Radiology Contrast Agents

- Diatrizoate meglumine sodium (Renografin)
- Iodized oil
- Iopanoic acid (Telepaque)
- Lipiodol
- Ipodate (Oragrafin)
- Iothalamate (Angio-Conray)
- Metrizamide (Omnipaque)

The decisions about medications and contrast agents are ones you will need to make with your doctor. Please make him or her aware if you have thyroid disease and if you are on thyroid medication. Ask if your medicine or contrast agent has iodine. If so, see if there are any safer alternatives.

DIETARY SUPPLEMENTS

Supplements are often a surprising source of iodine. Some have a lot of iodine because the manufacturers have added it, while others have too much because of poor quality control in the manufacturing.

Some supplements have iodine as the main ingredient. Common ones contain 12,500 to 50,000 mcg of iodine per tablet, and are completely unsafe. Thyroid support supplements nearly always contain added iodine. The amounts may be as low as 150 mcg, but are often in the thousands of micrograms. Nearly all multivitamins contain iodine. Bear in mind, though, that the amount of iodine in supplements is not well controlled in the manufacturing processes. In a recent study, 114 of the top brands of multivitamins were evaluated for their iodine content. Some were prescription prenatal supplements, and some were over-the-counter products. All had added iodine, with a labeled amount of iodine per serving.

Scientists suspected that some increases in thyroid disease could be due in part to higher than expected and fluctuating amounts of iodine in vitamins. The results shocked the scientists when they found the following:

- Not one single product contained the amount of iodine that was claimed on the label.
- The iodine in prescription vitamins was not better controlled than that in non-prescription vitamins.
- Kelp products were worse than those with potassium iodine.
- Some products had three times as much iodine as reported.

- Several products had 400 to 600 mcg of iodine when measured.[37]

The most cost- and time-effective choice is to use a thyroid-specific multivitamin in conjunction with a healthy diet. At DrChristianson.com, our Daily Reset Pack is a multivitamin, multimineral antioxidant packaged with additional calcium, magnesium, vitamin D, and certified low-iodine fish oil. It contains the full spectrum of nutrients needed by someone with thyroid disease, except for iron.

If someone does need iron, it is better to take it separately, at the same time but not within the same capsule. When iron is combined with other ingredients inside a multivitamin, it makes some of the minerals hard to absorb and can also inactivate the antioxidants. Unless you need more iron, you shouldn't be taking it in a supplement.

The action steps for supplements are simple:

1. As a bare minimum, avoid all supplements with any amount of labeled iodine.
2. Focus on supplements that are independently assayed for iodine status and share their test results.

INVISIBLE SOURCES COMBINED

You can see how any one of these invisible sources of iodine can be a problem. Imagine how easy it is to be exposed to more than one?

Each of the sources described here contributed significant amounts of iodine that could injure thyroid function. There's also a wide range of iodine in many of these sources, so it would be possible for people to have vastly different iodine intakes even if using similar items.

The following table shows how one's daily iodine intake could fluctuate on standard items and compares this to the amounts on the Thyroid Reset Diet. Remember, over 200 mcg of iodine per day can trigger thyroid disease, and under 100 mcg of it may reverse thyroid disease.

TYPICAL IODINE INTAKE

IODINE SOURCE	LOW	AVERAGE	HIGH	THYROID RESET DIET
Hair conditioner	0 mcg	100 mcg	540 mcg	0 mcg
Multivitamins	33 mcg	150 mcg	610 mcg	0 mcg (iodine-free multivitamin)
Salt	10 mcg	100 mcg	155 mcg	0 mcg (iodine-free salt)
Bread: 1 slice	2 mcg	300 mcg	1,174 mcg	0 mcg (no processed baked goods)
Milk: 16 ounces	166 mcg	200 mcg	720 mcg	15 mcg (low-iodine dairy)
Fish fillet: 100 grams	20 mcg	100 mcg	730 mcg	15 mcg (low-iodine seafood)
Eggs: 2 whole eggs	48 mcg	60 mcg	350 mcg	0 (no egg yolks)
Meat and poultry	0 mcg	50 mcg	91 mcg	15 mcg (low-iodine meat and poultry)
Whole grains and legumes	0 mcg	0 mcg	5 mcg	5 mcg
Fresh fruit	0 mcg	0 mcg	7 mcg	5 mcg
Vegetables	0 mcg	0 mcg	10 mcg	5 mcg
Nuts and seeds (unsalted)	0 mcg	0 mcg	3 mcg	0 mcg
Total daily intake	177 mcg	1,060 mcg	3,248 mcg	60 mcg

Sources: Pearce EN, Pino S, He X, Bazrafshan HR, Lee SL, Braverman LE. Sources of Dietary Iodine: Bread, Cows' Milk, and Infant Formula in the Boston Area. *J Clin Endocrinol Metab.* 2004;89(7):3421–3424. doi:10.1210/jc.2003-032002; Cowling T, Frey N. *Macrocyclic and Linear Gadolinium Based Contrast Agents for Adults Undergoing Magnetic Resonance Imaging: A Review of Safety.* Ottawa: Canadian Agency for Drugs and Technologies in Health, 2019

From this table, you can see why not everyone gets thyroid disease. Before even considering how different people respond to the same dose of iodine, it is clear that people using the same foods, supplements, and personal-care products can end up ingesting different amounts of iodine. Indeed, the person lucky enough to get all low-iodine items may not develop thyroid disease. But if someone does have thyroid disease, even an American diet that happens to have less iodine than is typical still may have enough iodine to prevent recovery.

Further, those people with average or high amounts of iodine in their chosen items could easily have thyroid disease triggered. The American Thyroid Association states that a daily intake above 1,100 mcg of iodine, even if short term, is unsafe and can trigger thyroid disease—for almost anyone.

Given all these invisible sources of iodine, you can understand why thyroid disease is on the rise. It also explains how easy it is to consume enough excess iodine to keep your thyroid disease going once it gets started. Now we'll take a look at how the Thyroid Reset Diet works to heal your thyroid.

Chapter Five

Thyroid Reset Diet

I know your thyroid journey has likely been a long, grueling, and frustrating process. So without further ado, let's get into the basics of the Thyroid Reset Diet. Here, you will learn how to regulate your iodine level so that your thyroid can work better. You will also learn how to eat to reduce your iodine intolerance. The more tolerant of iodine you become, the more freedom you will have in the Maintenance phase.

I made the diet easy to implement by giving you comprehensive food lists, menus, and recipes. You are welcome to follow the menus and recipes just as they are. You are also welcome to use these guidelines to adapt your own menus and recipes. In the food lists, I've grouped foods based on their iodine content.

Green Light foods have under 10 mcg of iodine per serving; these are safe to use without restriction during both the Reset phase and the Maintenance phase. Yellow Light foods have 10 to 50 mcg of iodine per serving. These are foods to be avoided during the Reset phase. During the Maintenance phase, you can add up to two servings of foods from the Yellow Light list daily. It is worth noting that Yellow Light foods often have specific serving sizes. That is because larger servings would contain more iodine, so stick with the specific portion, lest that cause a relapse of thyroid disease. Red Light foods often have over 50 mcg of iodine per serving. These are to be avoided as much as possible in the long term by anyone with thyroid disease.

No food categories have been excluded, but if you already have excluded some food for other reasons that are important to you, stick with that decision. If you are some version of vegan, gluten-free, or paleo, you'll find that there isn't much to change so as to regulate your iodine; you're already most of the way there.

As important as your thyroid is, this diet also supports your general health. It's what has been best documented to help you live longer and lower your risk for chronic disease. I can confirm that this plan is nutritionally complete.

THE TWO PHASES

THE RESET PHASE

Most of you will start here.

The goal of the Reset phase is to help your thyroid get rid of its excess iodine. This is the same plan as the one that has reversed thyroid disease in my clinical trials and that was used in the Case Stories mentioned throughout the book. You'll have to make some significant changes in your diet, but the results can be more than worth it. The Reset phase helps your body transition away from thyroid resistance and gives your thyroid its best chance to heal. The backlog of iodine trapped in the thyroid can make you feel like you're lacking thyroid hormones, even if you are taking enough. This could be the reason the thyroid medication did not restore your energy after your thyroid had slowed down.

The Reset phase may also restore thyroid function to the point that you may need less thyroid medication, or no medication at all. As a doctor, I always found it a blast when I got to call patients to tell them that they could stop their medication. That's what happens when the body is now working better than it has in years!

Plan to stay in the Reset phase for a minimum of three months. It is common in the first twenty-eight days to see some clear changes to your symptoms, and that should be encouraging. For example, if fatigue was your main symptom, watch how you function later in the day. Do you crash, or do you find yourself more able to pick up and prepare for the next day? How do you feel about exercise or physical tasks? That is, do you avoid them as much as before or have you started to look forward to them? If weight control was a struggle before, has it continued to increase or have you leveled off? How are your clothes fitting—any looser?

Hair loss takes the longest to resolve because hair grows so slowly. By the first month, though, it is common to notice that your shower drain is not filling up with hair as much. You may even see a few tiny new hairs growing in.

Even if you start to feel some wonderful changes taking place in the first month, give yourself the full three months in the Reset phase so that those improvements are consistent. At three months, you're cleared to progress to the Maintenance phase if one of the following is true:

- Your symptoms have improved.
- You no longer need thyroid medication.

Some people have thyroid disease that causes symptoms, but they aren't on medication. If that is your situation, and if your symptoms are resolved, you also should feel free to move to the Maintenance phase. However, it is still important to take the scheduled retests and make the follow-up visits with your doctor.

For those on thyroid medication, retesting and gentle adjustments under your doctors' care are essential. The decision to stop thyroid medication should be mutual. Most doctors who treat people with thyroid disease do not see their patients improve, and they are often unfamiliar with how to taper off medications in a way that keeps the patient's thyroid working. You can find recommendations for doctors who can help you taper on the resources page: www.thyroidresetdiet.com/resources.

If you have *not* seen your symptoms or blood levels improve after three months, see pages 87 and 88 about testing your iodine levels and your iodine individuality.

THE MAINTENANCE PHASE

Most of you will transition to this phase after completing the Reset. If you do not have thyroid disease, but would like to lower your risk of developing it, start here, with the Maintenance phase.

Think of Maintenance as a set of good eating habits to stick with in the long term. If you have had thyroid disease, you are susceptible to the effects of excess iodine. Even after your thyroid gets better, you run a higher risk that it will slow down in the future. The Maintenance phase helps you protect your thyroid against stress while opening up the option of up to two servings of Yellow Light foods per day.

THYROID RETESTING

You have some options for testing your thyroid. If you have easy access to lab tests and no financial barriers, the more data you gather, the better. If testing is more difficult for you, even just a TSH test can be helpful in assessing improvement. So, if you are on thyroid medication, or you have had abnormal thyroid levels on a recent blood test, retest your levels at the end of the Reset phase. The goal now is to see whether your levels are improving—it's okay if your numbers aren't perfect.

A full thyroid panel consists of a TSH, free T4, free T3, anti-TPO, anti-TG, and thyroglobulin. In general, the TSH is the main gauge of how much thyroid hormone is in your bloodstream. That is true regardless of whether the hormone comes from your thyroid or from thyroid medication.

A high TSH score means there is less hormone in your bloodstream, while a low TSH score means there is more. Most labs say that the normal range is between 0.4 and 4.5 IU/mL. Experts agree that this range is far too broad for many people, however. Which level is best can vary with pregnancy, age, cardiovascular health, and a history of thyroid cancer. Most otherwise healthy adults function best when the TSH is inside the normal range but on the lower end of it, such as 0.5 to 2.0 IU/mL.

The free T4 and free T3 measures tell more about how your liver is regulating the thyroid hormones. When the numbers are not consistent with the TSH, that suggests there are issues with hormone regulation, rather than problems with the amount of hormones. Anti-TPO, anti-TG, and thyroglobulin measures indicate whether there is autoimmune disease and give the rate of thyroid cell death.

How much do you need to test? If you have not had a full panel in a year, please do so. If you have had a full panel in the last year, you can also test just your TSH. The TSH does not tell you everything, but it is the first indicator when your thyroid levels start to improve. Remember, the TSH indicator is an opposite: if your thyroid is underactive, your TSH is too high. But at the end of three months on the Reset diet, it should be lower.

You can collect your TSH at home. There are special kits for collecting a dot of blood on a piece of paper, much like a home glucometer test. The piece of paper is then mailed to a laboratory, which analyzes the results and shares them with you and your doctor. You can learn more about home testing options at www.thyroidresetdiet.com/resources.

WHEN TO TEST

If your thyroid lab work was not done at the right time, the results could be off. This can make it look like things are not improving when they actually are. So, each time you get tested, follow these five rules:

1. Morning: Test your thyroid in the morning between 7 and 9 a.m.[1]
2. Fasting: Do your thyroid tests before drinking coffee or eating any food.[2,3,4]
3. Before taking thyroid medications: Do your thyroid tests before taking the morning dose of thyroid medication.[5,6]
4. No supplements for three days: Do your thyroid tests three days *after* your last dose of any supplements that contain biotin and *before* taking any other supplements for the day.[7]
5. Right time of your cycle: If you are a woman with a regular menstrual cycle, do your thyroid tests between days 1 and 9 of your period or between days 21 and 28. Do not take thyroid tests between days 10 and 20 of your cycle.[8,9]

If you start to have unusual symptoms and you are not due to get tested, reach out to your team and arrange for an early retest. It is also important to monitor any changes you may have had to the structure of your thyroid. If your thyroid doctor or radiologist suggests a certain time to repeat your ultrasound, do so as per their recommendation.

If your last ultrasound was normal, check with your thyroid doctor; each year, you should repeat the ultrasound or at least have your doctor examine your thyroid. If you have never had a thyroid ultrasound, then you are past due. Contact your thyroid doctor and get your baseline ultrasound done.

WHAT THE RESULTS MEAN

It does take the help of a thyroid specialist to definitively interpret your results, but here are some points to get you started.

The first indicator likely to change is your TSH. If your thyroid starts to make more hormones than it had before, the TSH goes lower. If you are on thyroid medication and your TSH moves below range (under 0.4 IU/mL), your doctor will likely need to change your prescription. If the TSH stays below range for too long, your thyroid's ability to heal diminishes and you become at risk for complications. These issues can still happen, even if you feel fine. It's rare, but there are some doctors who ignore a TSH below range. If your doctor does not treat that as a risk, seek out a thyroid specialist who is more cautious.

IODINE TESTING

If, after three months, you do not see the improvements in symptoms that you would have liked, also test your iodine levels. If they are still high, there must be some invisible source of iodine that is still getting into your system.

The only accurate test for iodine is the urinary iodine to creatinine ratio. That is, the amount of iodine in your urine is compared against the amount of a normal kidney protein, called creatinine. This urinary iodine to creatine ratio is tested with a random urine collection. The time of day is not important. This test can also be done at home and mailed in for convenience. Learn more about home testing options at www.thyroidresetdiet.com/resources. Many other iodine tests are available, but they are not accurate.

WHAT THE RESULTS MEAN

Iodine tests are not perfect, but they are helpful. The test will not tell you exactly how much iodine you are taking in, but it can reveal if you have reduced your iodine intake enough to help your thyroid.

The urinary test results are reported as a mcg of iodine per gram of creatinine, abbreviated as mcg/G. If your levels are over 100 mcg/G, you have not eliminated enough hidden sources of iodine. The goal is to be under 100 mcg/G. The higher your scores are above this range, the more iodine you are still ingesting.

Many people do not see improvements on the Thyroid Reset Diet until their iodine levels are under 100 mcg/G. If this happens to you, revisit Chapter Four about invisible iodine to see where you might be getting the iodine. Once you have adjusted your diet, you can retest your urine as soon as two weeks later to confirm that you are now within the right range.

IODINE INDIVIDUALITY AND IODINE INTOLERANCE

As you begin the Reset phase, it is worth knowing that people respond differently to iodine regulation. That is, some respond quickly, others take more time, and some do not respond at all. This fact ties into why not everyone gets thyroid disease, even if his or her iodine levels are not right. I call these differences "iodine individuality" and "iodine intolerance."

Iodine individuality is how your body is genetically prone to respond to iodine. People have different responses, and they cannot be changed. If your body is taking a little longer to respond to the diet, this may be why. Researchers think that such lasting differences relate to our ancestral exposure to iodine. If we go back far enough in human history, we find that locally grown food was not just a good idea, it was the only option.

For our ancestors near the ocean, the soils were rich in iodine and therefore most of the gathered or cultivated food was as well. In addition, seafood was a big part of the diet. Over generations, these people adapted to a higher intake of iodine. Earlier, I described how the thyroid has to absorb iodine into itself. Our coastal ancestors needed a weaker absorbing action or else they would overload their thyroids. If they suddenly were in a low-iodine food environment, they may not have fared well, but their food environment rarely changed abruptly.

We also had ancestors who lived far inland, at high elevations or near large bodies of fresh water. These people were in low-iodine food environments. They needed a stronger absorbing action to transfer every speck of iodine from their bloodstreams into their thyroid glands. Some areas had so little naturally occurring iodine that there were high rates of goiter or cretinism. Yet if these people suddenly had a high intake of iodine, their thyroid glands would have been overloaded with iodine in no time.

We can't change our iodine individuality; it is largely fixed by genetics. In contrast, our current health can make us more sensitive to iodine for reasons we *can* change. I call this our level of iodine intolerance.

The biggest known variable here is one's selenium status. Selenium is an essential mineral for humans. If you are low in selenium, your body loses the ability to form glutathione within the thyroid or to tolerate the free radicals generated from iodine. Having enough selenium helps you maintain good thyroid function across a broader range of iodine intake. Other minerals that play important roles in iodine tolerance are iron and zinc. Those who have too little of these minerals are unable to produce some of the enzymes involved in regulating the thyroid hormones. That's why the Thyroid Reset Diet comprises foods that are especially dense in these important minerals. If you get appropriate amounts of these minerals from whole foods, you can mend an iodine intolerance. Then your thyroid will have a better chance of getting healthy, even with some minor iodine fluctuations.

You'll find out how to do that in just a few pages!

GETTING STARTED

In the Thyroid Reset Diet, all foods are divided into three categories: Green Light, Yellow Light, and Red Light. In the Reset phase, you only eat foods from the Green Light list.

Chapter Seven has the iodine content for the detailed food lists in these three categories. The food lists are derived mostly from the FDA's *Total Diet Study: Elemental Results Summary Statistics*.[10] I supplemented their list with results from additional large databases and research studies so as to include more options for foods like nuts, seafood, vegetables, fruits, grain products, and sea vegetables.[11,12]

If you would like more details on these sources, download my iodine content spreadsheet. Alas, it is much too big to fit into this book!

It includes the mcg of iodine per serving for each food, sorted by category, iodine range, and maximum iodine per sample. You can find it at www.thyroidresetdiet.com/resources.

The default serving size for foods on the Thyroid Reset Diet is 100 grams. This is just over 3 ounces in weight. Some foods, like beverages, have a larger serving size; others, like anchovies, are smaller serving sizes. That is, the serving sizes fit typical amounts used; if this is not the case, there is a note indicating the change made and why.

GREEN LIGHT FOODS

These foods have negligible amounts of iodine, regardless of serving size. At most, they may have 10 mcg of iodine per serving size, without significant variation from sample to sample. Examples of these are brown rice, chicken breast, kale, onion, garlic, ginger, sesame oil, and soy sauce.

These Green Light foods can be freely eaten on both the Reset and the Maintenance phases. Do bear in mind, of course, that there may be other reasons to limit these foods. For example, white rice, olive oil, and almonds are all Green Light foods, yet if they were added to the diet in unlimited quantities, they could lead to weight gain, which causes a strain on the thyroid.

YELLOW LIGHT FOODS

These foods usually have 10 to 50 mcg of iodine per serving, without much variation from sample to sample. In the Maintenance phase, two servings of these foods can be eaten per day from any category. For example, if you have a 1-ounce serving of Swiss cheese on a given day, you would not also have salmon that same day. Other Yellow Light foods include egg yolks and salmon. Note that in amounts above the serving size, all Yellow Light foods should be considered Red Light foods, or not permitted.

RED LIGHT FOODS

These are foods that often have over 50 mcg of iodine per serving—in many cases, even several thousand mcg per serving. These foods are to be avoided in both the Reset and the Maintenance phases. Examples include kelp, ice cream, commercial bread, and codfish.

There are lots of good food options in the Green and Yellow categories. Also, don't assume that you can't ever have any food from the Red Light category, just that they are best avoided whenever possible.

For some, dietary changes seem overwhelming, so going slowly at first feels better. Others are comfortable diving right in. Both approaches can work, as long as you're getting rid of those hidden sources of iodine.

Here is a one-week suggested transition into the diet. If you are eager to start right away, feel free follow all these steps your first day, but make sure you complete each step!

ONE-WEEK TIERED TRANSITION

Before starting the diet, shop for the Thyroid Reset essentials listed here. If you are vegan or following the autoimmune paleo (AIP) diet, feel free to ignore the suggestions for any food categories that you already avoid. Eat as you have been doing so up until this point, except for the Daily Step for each day.

THYROID RESET ESSENTIALS

- **KOSHER SALT** You do not have to stop using salt or skimp on its use. You just want to be sure you are using salt that won't add iodine. Kosher salt is the easiest choice. If you love sea salt, try Celtic's light gray sea salt. It comes in fine and coarse versions, and both are fine. Other brands of sea salt or other products made by Celtic may not be low in iodine.

- **DAIRY** Obtain dairy substitutes to replace the dairy foods in your diet. There are so many non-dairy, plant-based options for milk, yogurt, cheese, ice cream, and butter. I do like those fortified with vitamin D and calcium. Some of the plant-based milks even have extra protein added. Avoid products with carrageenan.

    Good options include flax milk, coconut yogurt, Smart Balance spread, and vegan cheese. If these foods are new to you, buy several different brands so you can try them and find which you like best. When you get home, discard the dairy products made from cows' milk. If you use eggs, buy liquid egg whites as their replacement.

- **WHOLE GRAINS AND LEGUMES** Great options include brown rice, buckwheat, and steel-cut oats. If you like soft homemade flatbread, pick up some all-purpose flour. If you are gluten-free, get some gluten-free all-purpose flour.

THE FIRST WEEK

DAY 1: COSMETICS

Chapter Four discussed how you could be getting large amounts of iodine through your cosmetics. Look through your lotions and conditioners and find any with hidden iodine. Compare the list of ingredients in Chapter Four against the ingredient lists for your products. If you find any that have iodine-containing ingredients, it is time to shop for substitutes. Thankfully, you have plenty of products available that are iodine-free and that will work as well, if not better. You can find a current list of cosmetic brands that avoid iodine-containing ingredients on www.thyroidresetdiet.com/resources.

DAY 2: SUPPLEMENTS

For many people, supplements may be their highest source of iodine. Some iodine pills by themselves contain 50,000 mcg. Given that over 200 mcg per day can be a problem for some people, an iodine pill by itself can have 125 times more iodine than is safe, not counting other food sources.

Gather all your pills and check the nutritional facts panels. If any bottles list iodine in any amount, put them in the discard pile. Of those that are left, check the ingredient lists. Any that have the word "iodine" or "iodo" in the ingredient list should also be discarded. Of those that are left, check the ingredient lists for kelp, whey, egg, or "sea" anything. Discard any that have those words.

What should you replace these with? You may need some supplements to address specific concerns, and some nutrients are good for almost any adult. If you were taking supplements for a specific concern, like digestive health, hair, or inflammation, work with a healthcare practitioner to find iodine-free options. Ask your healthcare practitioner to tell you how long to take them and how to be sure they are working. I say that because far too many people add pills to their day because they seem like a good idea at the time and they end up taking them indefinitely. Also, taking a large number of pills may cause side effects that you would not expect from taking any of the pills individually. Don't take pills that are not essential.

For essential nutrients, people prone to thyroid disease often have needs that are distinct from the general population. Vitamins that might work just fine for anyone else might not work well for you. Yet you want to get all the essential vitamins, minerals, and fatty acids on a daily basis. This should include water-soluble vitamins like vitamin C, thiamin, riboflavin, niacin, vitamin B6, folate, vitamin B12, biotin, pantothenic acid; and fat-soluble vitamins like vitamin A, vitamin D, vitamin K, vitamin E; plus all essential minerals, including calcium, magnesium, zinc, selenium, copper, manganese, chromium, molybdenum, and boron. The B vitamins should be in their active form, such as pyridoxal 5-phosphate for B6 and methyl cobalamin for B12. Some vitamins should have a range of isomers as found in food; for example, vitamin K should include K1, K2, MK-6, MK-7, and MK-9.

The main things to avoid are iodine and folic acid. Folic acid is a synthetic form of folate that some people cannot process owing to their gene variations. These variations are called MTHF-R, and they are present in over 99 percent of those with thyroid disease.

For those who want an easy option, I've created a forum Daily Reset Pack that takes all these considerations into account. It also has fish oil that is confirmed as low in iodine and a full dose of calcium, magnesium, and vitamin D. Finally, there are bonus nutrients including quercetin, trans resveratrol, and benfotiamine that have been shown to help the body's ability to regulate thyroid hormones. You can find more about it and other supplement options at www.thyroidresetdiet.com/resources.

DAY 3: SALT AND SEA VEGETABLES

Now you get to make use of your recent shopping trip! Time to try out the new salt. If you follow any chefs, nearly all of them use kosher salt. It turns out that added iodine leaves a bitter taste that is obvious to those with sensitive palates. See if you notice the difference.

Next up is sea vegetables. They can be foods onto themselves, or they can be ingredients in other foods. When used as foods, these come dried in quart-sized plastic bags. The most common products are dulse, kombu, wakame, nori, and hijiki. Discard these products. They're also commonly found in Asian dried seasonings. You will see toasted nori or kelp mixed with salt and toasted sesame seeds, for example. Look over all your seasonings and spices and discard those with for kelp, nori, kombu, agar, or dulse.

At this point, you have taken three large steps to plummet your toxic iodine intake, and you have not even had to change a single meal!

DAY 4: DAIRY

Today you get to start using your plant-based dairy products. If you like milk as a beverage, oat milk can be a good substitute. For cooking, flax, oat, almond, and soy milk can work well without overpowering the recipe's flavor. Non-dairy yogurts are easy substitutes, although they are usually lower in protein; you may need to add another serving of the protein food to compensate. There are some great non-dairy cheeses out there—or you could easily make them at home.

DAY 5: GRAINS

Today is the day to make use of iodine-free grain products. Throw out any commercial breads or baked goods. If you mostly have grain products as a side dish, start with the Basic Brown Rice on page 228. If you used bread for wraps, sandwiches, or toast, try the Easy Flatbread on page 226. I like to make double batches of flatbread and freeze it.

DAY 6: EGGS

If you use eggs in cooking, egg whites are a perfect substitute. Use ¼ cup of liquid egg whites for each large egg in a recipe. Sprinkle in a few shakes of dried turmeric and paprika, and you will even have the color of yolky scrambled eggs and omelets. If you have leftover whole eggs, just toss the yolks. Be sure to try the Egg White Omelet on page 168.

DAY 7: PLANNING AHEAD

You have already taken the main steps! Today, take some time to plan your next week's menu. Look over the QuickStart Guide (page 104) and the Week 1 meal plan. If you prefer to use your own recipes, review the food lists and the meal assembly guide.

OTHER DIETARY CONSIDERATIONS

The Thyroid Reset Diet is structured so that you receive the optimal amount of iodine to improve or stabilize your thyroid function. But there are other dietary factors that are important for thyroid health, so they've been built into the diet as well. These include certain foods, macronutrient ratios, micronutrient sufficiency, and proportional intake of certain food groups.

To be clear, none of these other factors have as much compelling evidence as does iodine. Nonetheless, they have some degree of importance and therefore have been included as part of the Thyroid Reset Diet. Two specific food types are helpful to include on a regular basis: vegetables and Brazil nuts.

VEGETABLES

In a large study of over 10,000 participants, high vegetable intake was shown to improve thyroid autoimmunity more than any factor besides regulating iodine.[13] The vegetables counted in the study included leafy greens like spinach, root vegetables like onions, flowering vegetables like broccoli, and legumes like lentils.

Make your goal to eat 5 or more cups of vegetables per day. Drop 1 or 2 cups of spinach into your morning smoothie, add some beans to your salad for lunch, have another salad or a main dish with vegetables for dinner, and you're there.

Every day, eat at least 1 cup each of the following:

- Leafy greens, like kale, collards, romaine, spinach, arugula, and chard
- Alliums, like onions, leeks, garlic, shallots, scallions, and chives
- Cruciferous vegetables, like broccoli, cauliflower, cabbage, bok choy, Brussels sprouts, and turnips

BRAZIL NUTS

Brazil nuts seem to have unique benefits for good thyroid function. Part of that may be because they are rich in selenium, and selenium makes the thyroid tolerant of a broader range of iodine. But Brazil nuts have been shown to help thyroid function more than one would expect from their selenium content alone.[14]

They contain a version of selenium that is safer than the type in many supplements. The safest chemical form of selenium is one called selenomethionine. The human body can safely store selenomethionine in blood proteins and use it as needed; it is also easily excreted by the body in cases of excess. Some people warn of the dangers of selenium overdose from Brazil nuts. However, there have been no documented cases of selenium toxicity from Brazil nuts. In Brazil nuts, 75 to 90 percent of the selenium is in the form of selenomethionine.[15]

Brazil nuts have a neutral flavor and are easy to add to pretty much anything. Eat them as a snack, blend them into your smoothie, or add them to hot cereal. You can even chop them up and lightly toast them to add to stir-fry dishes.

MACRONUTRIENTS

In addition to regulating iodine intake, the Thyroid Reset Diet contains a balance of fats, carbohydrates, and proteins. Data have shown that diets extremely high or low in any one macronutrient may be less effective than diets in which the micronutrients are all represented.

FATS

Several lines of evidence show that thyroid-healthy diets favor the essential fats found in nuts, seeds, and low-iodine seafood over the nonessential fats found in lard, butter, and processed meats.[16]

CARBOHYDRATES

Many people have gotten used to thinking about carbohydrates as best minimized because they may raise insulin production. Yet we now know that insulin is essential to activate the thyroid hormones.

Too much insulin can be a bad thing, but when insulin is too low, the body goes into many adaptations of starvation. One of these adaptations is to slow the metabolism down by blocking the thyroid hormones. It turns out that even if you are not starving or losing weight, too little carbohydrate in the diet can block thyroid hormones. Controlled studies have shown that having adequate carbohydrates is essential to maintain T3 levels.[17]

Along with changes to the metabolism, suppression of T3 from low-carbohydrate diets can speed up the rate of muscle loss. Studies have shown that even when someone is eating enough food to maintain weight, low-carb diets that lower T3 have increased muscle loss by 53 percent.[18]

If you are not trying to lose weight, you can likely maintain thyroid function, at least in the short term, on 70 grams of carbohydrate per day, or as little as 40 percent of total calories. That can be several smaller servings or one larger serving. If you are attempting to lose weight, your thyroid may be even more sensitive to a low-carbohydrate diet.[19,20]

The amounts of carbohydrate used in studies that improved T3 metabolism ranged from as low as 40 percent of calories to as high as 55 percent. This range is roughly on a par with the amounts associated with the best overall health.

The healthiest sources of carbohydrates are vegetables like yams, squash, turnips, or potatoes; legumes like pinto beans, lentils, or peas; or whole grains like quinoa, buckwheat, or brown rice. If your diet is not restricted, using a variety of carbohydrate sources is ideal because each offers a different type of fiber.

PROTEIN

Protein is helpful for good thyroid function. Diets that are too low in protein can slow the production of thyroid hormones. That is, diets with less protein cause an elevation of thyroid-binding globulin, the carrier compound that neutralizes the thyroid hormones. Low-protein diets may also cause more harm from exposure to excessive iodine.[21] Protein requirements are likely more critical to thyroid function for women during weight loss or dieting.[22]

Considering these points, how much protein is best? A good rule of thumb is to eat a gram of protein per pound of lean body weight each day. For example, if a woman is 140 pounds and 25 percent is body fat, she has 35 pounds of fat (140 × 0.25 = 35). Therefore, she has roughly 105 pounds of lean body mass (140 − 35 = 105).

She does not need this much protein to prevent protein deficiency. But on much less than this, she may lose muscle mass, which slows her metabolism and can suppress her thyroid.

Protein is worth thinking about as grams per day rather than as a percentage of calories because even if you eat less food, you still need just as much protein.

MACRONUTRIENT RATIOS

When we put all the macronutrients together, the best ratios of them for the Thyroid Reset Diet are as follows:

- Protein: roughly 1 gram per pound of lean body mass
- Fats: 10 to 40 percent of calories
- Carbohydrates: 40 to 55 percent of calories

Note that the ranges are broadest for fats and carbohydrates. So, how do you choose? For most people, the difference is not important if they don't overeat and they choose mostly unprocessed foods. All studies to date have shown that, once you control for protein intake, low-carb or low-fat diets aren't necessary for weight loss or general health.[23]

MICRONUTRIENTS

Every known vitamin and mineral plays some helpful role in the production or use of the thyroid hormones or in helping avoid autoimmunity. Some, like iodine and selenium, are central to thyroid function. A few others that often are lacking and do directly impact the disease process include iron and zinc. Diets can be either deficient in iron and zinc or have poor absorption.

SELENIUM SUPPLEMENTATION

It appears that selenium supplements may offer benefits to thyroid function that are distinct from those of dietary selenium. As one such example, selenium supplementation has been shown in three placebo-controlled clinical human trials to reduce thyroid antibodies. The average reduction studied over six months ranged from 25 to 55 percent for thyroid peroxidase antibodies, with doses ranging from 100 to 200 mcg of selenium daily. Selenium supplementation has also been shown to reduce abnormal findings on thyroid ultrasound studies.[24]

One can get too much selenium, and its toxicity is like that of lead poisoning. An intake consistently above 400 mcg per day can produce symptoms like diarrhea, fatigue, hair loss, joint pain, and others.[25] Selenium toxicity has emerged as a side effect from poorly produced liquid mineral supplements that contained hundreds of times the labeled amount.[26]

Along with selenium, other micronutrients can help the thyroid by improving its iodine regulating enzymes. You can read more about deiodinase support at www.thyroidresetdiet.com/resources.

If you eat the recommended amount of Brazil nuts and take 100 mcg of selenium in supplement form, you don't have to worry about overconsumption of selenium.

IRON

Iron is an important consideration for the Thyroid Reset Diet, for several reasons.

Women who are menstruating, or were in recent years, are prone to iron deficiency from the blood loss of menstruation. Some have even speculated that this may be one of the reasons for the higher rate of thyroid disease among women. When iron is even a little bit low, the thyroid is more sensitive to iodine fluctuations.[27]

Iron is found in plant foods and animal foods, although the chemical types of iron are different. Animal foods have a version called heme iron, since the iron found in them is bound to the protein hemoglobin. Plant foods contain non-heme iron. Both are absorbable, but the percentages differ.

Those who do not consume animal protein can maintain their iron status, but if they have factors causing malabsorption, they can be more easily at risk for iron deficiency. Some of the better sources of iron are avoided in the Thyroid Reset Diet because of their iodine content. These include clams, egg yolks, and some types of fish.

The Thyroid Reset Diet supplies iron from:

- Dark poultry
- Kidney beans
- Leafy green vegetables
- Lentils
- Lima beans
- Navy beans
- Red meat
- Tempeh
- White beans

If you have or suspect an iron deficiency, medical guidance is essential. Some people need iron supplements in addition to high-iron foods. Some need iron infusions in addition to iron supplements. Many are simply unable to improve their thyroid symptoms until their iron deficiency is lessened. Work with your doctor to check your levels. If they are low, increase the iron in your diet or through supplementation.

ZINC

Zinc is a mineral essential to the body for numerous chemical reactions, including thyroid hormone production, immune cell regulation, ovarian function, detoxification pathways, tissue production, and more. People with thyroid disease are more likely to be low in zinc.[28]

A study was done to see if zinc supplementation could improve thyroid function. In it, sixty-eight women with hypothyroidism were divided into four groups. One group received a supplement containing 30 mg of zinc and 200 mcg of selenium, one received a zinc + placebo pill; one received a selenium + placebo pill; and the final group only took a placebo. After twelve weeks, their thyroid levels were compared to those measured before the study began. Those taking selenium and zinc saw improvement in all measured thyroid markers, but none of the other groups did. Yet none was deficient in zinc, nor did any see their zinc blood levels change.[29]

This is an example of how nutrients can help even those who are not deficient in those nutrients. That is why the Thyroid Reset Diet encourages supplementation in addition to the diet for all with thyroid disease. Eat at least one rich dietary source of zinc and get at least 10 mg of chelated zinc in your supplementation.

The Thyroid Reset Diet supplies zinc from the following:

- Dark meat poultry
- Green peas
- Hemp seeds
- Lentils
- Lima beans
- Oats
- Potatoes
- Pumpkin seeds
- Red meat
- Shiitake mushrooms
- Spinach

CALCIUM

Calcium intake is important, for two main reasons: thyroid disease can create a greater need for calcium, and low-iodine diets may provide too little calcium.

One of the metabolic issues common to thyroid disease is an inability to prevent the formation of calcified tissues. These can form in the blood vessels, joints, kidneys, tendons, or elsewhere in the body.[30,31] The solution is to include plenty of low-iodine high-calcium foods in the diet and to supplement with soluble plant-derived versions of calcium, like dicalcium malate, calcium citrate, and calcium lactate.

Adults should strive to get roughly 400 to 500 mg of calcium from combined sources.[32] Those on high-dairy diets commonly consume much more calcium, but their bodies excrete much of it.[33] Possible sources of calcium include foods such as those listed here, plus calcium supplements and calcium-fortified foods.

The best food options include:

- Dried figs—241 mg per 8 figs
- Kale—180 mg per 2 cups
- Chia seeds—179 mg per 2 tablespoons
- Sesame seeds—176 mg per 2 tablespoons
- White beans—161 mg per cooked 1 cup
- Broccoli rabe—100 mg per 1 cup
- Edamame—98 mg per 1 cup
- Almonds—97 mg per ¼ cup
- Collard greens—84 mg per 1 cup
- Okra—82 mg per 1 cup

When you look through this food list, you will realize that getting 500 mg of calcium per day is possible, but may take some thought and planning.

For those who may be running low on calcium, it is best to add roughly 300 mg of dicalcium malate. I formulated our Daily Reset Pack to have 350 mg total of dicalcium malate. This type of calcium is one of the best for those with thyroid disease. Get at least 400 mg of calcium from your diet, then add 200 to 350 mg of plant-derived calcium supplements to lower the risk of bone thinning.

QuickStart Guide

I know you've just processed a lot of information, so the Thyroid Reset Diet is condensed here, in four basic rules:

1. **SALT**   Use kosher salt, canning salt, or Celtic brand light gray sea salt. Avoid iodized salt, unbranded sea salt, and pink Himalayan salt.
2. **FOOD**   Eat all fresh vegetables, fruits, unsalted nuts and seeds, fresh meat and poultry; whole grains and legumes; egg whites; and vegan dairy and egg substitutes that do not have carrageenan or other seaweed extracts. Avoid highly processed foods, dairy, egg yolks, most seafood, and all sea vegetables. Eat two to four Brazil nuts per day. See food lists for details.

    Also, eat 5 or more cups of vegetables per day. Eat a wide variety of vegetables. Each day, include at least one serving of greens (spinach, romaine, arugula, chard, and more); alliums (onions, garlic, shallots, scallions, and chives); cruciferous vegetables (broccoli, cauliflower, cabbage, bok choy, and more).
3. **SUPPLEMENTS AND MEDICATIONS**   Use an iodine-free multivitamin with selenium, zinc, and folate. Avoid all vitamins and medications containing iodine or folic acid.

    Note: Thyroid medications do contain iodine. This is one more reason that people on thyroid medication need to be mindful of their total iodine intake. Because the iodine in thyroid medications is bound up with hormones, it's important to reduce iodine from other sources. Unless a medication's dose is too high, lowering the dose prematurely does not help the thyroid heal.
4. **COSMETICS**   For conditioner, sunscreen, skin cream, and face lotion, avoid all with PVP or other iodine extracts.

CAN VEGAN OR AIP DIETS WORK?

There are many anecdotal reports of people improving their thyroid function on autoimmune paleo (AIP) or vegan diets. Assuming some of the anecdotes are true, how can these diets work when they are different from each other and different from the Thyroid Reset Diet? Even though these diets are all different, they are often naturally low in iodine. Many people who start one of these diets lower their iodine intake significantly. Here are some estimates to illustrate my point. I found some popular menus for the Standard American Diet (SAD), vegan diets, and the AIP diet. For each, I calculated the average iodine content for the day. The differences are striking.

Here is the amount of iodine you could easily get on a typical SAD diet. Using conservative estimates, this comes to over 500 mcg of iodine per day.

STANDARD AMERICAN DIET				
FOOD	SERVING	WEIGHT IN GRAMS	AVERAGE MCG OF IODINE PER GRAM	TOTAL
Iodized table salt	½ teaspoon	3	56.80	142.00
Breakfast*				
Eggs	1 egg	80	0.60	47.76
Bagel	1 bagel	100	0.42	41.90
Milk	8 ounces	240	0.40	96.72
Orange juice	8 ounces	240	0.06	13.68
Lunch†				
Bread	2 slices	100	0.86	86.00
Cheese	1 slice	30	0.45	13.44
Ham	3 ounces	100	0.00	0.30
Mayo	1 tablespoon	15	0.03	0.42
Clam chowder	1 cup	240	0.26	61.44

Dinner[#]				
Tortilla	2 tortillas	60	0.01	0.66
Beef	3 ounces	100	0.05	5.00
Rice	½ cup	200	0.00	0.20
Cheese	2 ounces	60		
Sour cream	½ ounce	15	0.37	5.54
Pinto beans	½ cup	200	0.00	0.00
Salsa	¼ cup	50	0.05	2.65
Snack				
Candy bar	1 bar	100	0.64	63.60
Apple	1 piece	100	0.00	0.00
			Day's intake	581.31

[*] Forbes J. What Do Americans Eat for Breakfast? Quora. November 24, 2011
[†] Pannell E. What Do Americans Eat For Lunch? Quora. March 15, 2015
[#] Hunt K. What's for Dinner: America's Meals from 1900 to 2000. Thrillist

Here is a daily AIP menu from a popular website. The day's iodine total was under 70 mcg!

AIP DAILY MENU				
FOOD	SERVING	WEIGHT IN GRAMS	AVERAGE MCG OF IODINE PER GRAM	TOTAL
Sea salt	½ teaspoon	3	20.00	50.00
Breakfast				
Ground beef	¼ pound	113	0.05	5.65
Cabbage	2 ounces	60	0.01	0.72
Lunch				
Smoked salmon	2 ounces	60	0.15	9.12
Bacon	½ slice	30	0.00	0.06
Basil	1 tablespoon	5	0.00	0.00

Leaf lettuce	2 cups	120	0.01	0.84
Olive oil	1 teaspoon		0.04	0.00
Dinner				
Ground turkey	¼ pound	113	0.00	0.11
Duck fat	1 tablespoon	15	0.00	0.00
Olive oil	1 teaspoon	5	0.04	0.20
Carrots	3 large	100	0.00	0.30
			Day's intake	**66.70**

Source: Etesin UM, Ite AE, Ukpong EJ, Ikpe EE, Ubong UU, Isotuk IG. Comparative Assessment of Iodine Content of Commercial Table Salt Brands Available in Nigerian Market. *Am J Hypertens Res.* 2017;4(1):9–14. doi:10.12691/ajhr-4-1-2

If you are already committed to AIP principles, the Thyroid Reset Diet will be easy!

Going forward, you should include as many of the AIP-approved thyroid support foods as you can. You should also make the switch from sea salt to non-iodized salt, limit consumption of high-iodine seafood, and avoid sea vegetables. Also, make sure your supplements and medications are free of iodine.

VEGAN DIETS AND THYROID DISEASE

Vegan diets are typically lower in iodine, and vegans may have lower levels of urinary iodine.[34] This is likely why published studies have shown that people on vegan diets have lower risks of developing thyroid disease, but this benefit is not shared with ovo-lacto vegetarians, who include eggs and dairy in their diet.[35] Since eggs and dairy are among the highest iodine sources in the diet, this distinction suggests that the inclusion of healthy plant foods and the reduction of dietary iodine are likely part of the reason vegan diets seem to help thyroid function.

Here is a day's menu from a popular vegan diet website, with my addition of iodine content. It comes in under 50 mcg per day.

VEGAN MENU				
FOOD	SERVING	WEIGHT IN GRAMS	AVERAGE MCG OF IODINE PER GRAM	TOTAL
Himalayan salt	1 teaspoon	5	5.00	25.00
Breakfast				
Tempeh bacon	1 slice	14	0.35	5.00
Mushrooms	1 ounce	30	0.00	0.18
Avocado	2 ounces	60	0.00	0.00
Arugula	2 cups	150	0.00	0.00
Lunch				
Whole-grain pasta	2 ounces	60	0.00	0.00
Pinto beans	½ cup	120	0.00	0.00
Lettuce	2 cups	150	0.00	0.00
Cauliflower	1 cup	64	0.00	0.00
Dinner				
Chickpeas	½ cup	120	0.04	5.00
Avocado	2 ounces	60	0.00	0.00
Tomato	2 ounces	60	0.00	0.00
Snacks				
Popcorn	3 cups	30	0.01	0.27
Kale chips, homemade	1 cup	15	0.00	0.00
Peanuts	¼ cup	40	0.15	6.00
Raisins	¼ cup	36	0.00	0.00
			Day's intake	41.45

Source: Link R. A Complete Vegan Meal Plan and Sample Menu. Healthline. Accessed August 4, 2019

If you are vegan and starting the Thyroid Reset Diet, you're already on your way with some solid guidelines. As far as further things to consider, be sure to avoid baked goods and processed foods possibly made with iodized salt. Also, look out for sea veggies and the iodine that can be in vitamins and medications. Be sure to add the recommended thyroid support foods, like Brazil nuts. Finally, look over the discussion about macronutrients. Vegans do not get protein deficient, but some fall below the amounts best for optimal thyroid function.

WHAT IF YOU'RE NOT PERFECT?

Any amount of unnecessary iodine that you can avoid will make things that much easier on your thyroid. In many of the studies, some people saw improved thyroid function even if they were not as thorough as others at avoiding iodine. Don't let the perfect be the enemy of the good.

It is entirely possible to polish off a meal without thinking it through. It is also possible to realize that a particular food is not in your best interests, and eat it anyway. Your benefits will be a function of the net reductions you make over the weeks to come. Your choices do matter, but don't think you will have to start from scratch if there's a single mishap.

Once you have seen your symptoms clear up and your thyroid is working better, it gets easier. The Maintenance phase includes suggestions that will help you keep your thyroid healthy over the long term.

Chapter Six

The Maintenance Phase

You made it! Think of Maintenance as your graduation. You've reset your thyroid by clearing out the excess iodine. For many people, this will mean they feel fine and they no longer need thyroid medication. For others, this will mean they feel better on a reasonable dose of stable medication.

Most people should be able to reach this point in three or more months. Right now, you should be feeling as well as you did before your thyroid disease started, if not better. If you have any remaining symptoms, they should be getting better. If you're still suffering, though, I've got a resource you can easily access: the Personalized Thyroid Plan. You can learn more about it at www.thyroidresetdiet.com/resources.

Moving forward, it is best to check in with your medical team at least twice per year, and make sure all your levels are stable and healthy. If you have had an abnormal ultrasound in the past, it is a good idea to repeat the examination at least once annually to make sure no negative changes are occurring with regard to the structure of your thyroid.

If you are not on thyroid medication, you should still recheck your levels at least once per year. Those who have had thyroid disease and have gone into remission still have a higher chance of redeveloping thyroid disease. It is also possible to develop a disease of a different type. Those who are in remission from Hashimoto's, for example, have a higher risk of developing Graves' disease or subclinical hypothyroidism.

It is also important to stay mindful of regulating your iodine intake. Continue being diligent about finding the invisible sources and staying clear of processed baked goods. Don't let your guard down and start consuming too many dairy foods. Be sure to check ingredients on any new personal-care products.

THE MAINTENANCE DIET

All the recipes and the meal plans for the Reset phase can be used during the Maintenance phase. You can still freely use the Green Light foods, and you still want to avoid the Red Light foods. The difference here is that you can add up to two servings of Yellow Light foods each day.

Please note that this addition is for the total number of foods, not the number of foods per category. For example, if you already added two Yellow Light dairy foods on a given day, you would not add Yellow Light seafood that same day. As you transition to your Maintenance diet, you still want to focus on eating unprocessed foods and keeping tabs on your food quantity.

FOCUS ON UNPROCESSED FOODS

The Thyroid Reset Diet focuses on unprocessed and minimally processed foods, for a variety of reasons. Besides improving thyroid health, diets rich in unprocessed food have been shown to fill you up faster,[1] lower your risk of developing chronic disease,[2] and lower your possibility of early mortality.[3]

Several different systems categorize how processed certain foods are. All are helpful and all have a few limitations, but I've simplified these to create the following system:

- Unprocessed foods are whole foods as found in nature, with no processing beyond cooking, fermentation, sprouting, and separating edible from inedible portions.

Some examples of unprocessed food are:

- Vegetables—All fresh and frozen vegetables, fermented vegetables.
- Fruit—All fresh and frozen fruit.
- Dairy—Milk, yogurt.
- Legumes—Cooked legumes.
- Grains—Sprouted whole grains, cooked whole grains. Examples include whole-grain brown rice, quinoa, and buckwheat.
- Nuts and seeds—All raw nuts and seeds.
- Seafood—All fresh or frozen cuts of finfish, shellfish, crustaceans, mollusks, and bivalves. Examples include salmon fillets, steamed clams, and fresh oysters.
- Meats and poultry—All fresh or frozen cuts of beef, pork, lamb, chicken, turkey, and other types of poultry.
- Salt—Iodine-free land salt, such as canning (pickling salt); possibly higher in iodine are sea salt, Himalayan salt.

If 80 to 90 percent of your diet comes from unprocessed foods, you'll be fine. Try to cut out or substitute any highly processed foods from your diet.

Even when you are eating whole foods, quantities still matter. You likely know that thyroid disease can lead to weight gain. New research has shown that being overweight can also lead to thyroid disease.[4] As you eat to keep your thyroid healthy, bear in mind that too much of the right foods can be just as harmful to your thyroid as eating the wrong foods.

FOOD FOR THE MAINTENANCE PHASE

Since you have more iodine tolerance (see page 88) by this point, you can now mix things up a bit more. For instance, if you have no other reasons to avoid dairy, egg yolks, or seafood, you now have more latitude in your diet. It is easy to take any of the recipes for the Reset phase and adapt them for the Maintenance phase. During the Maintenance phase you can include up to two of the Yellow Light foods. Here are some ways to modify the Thyroid Reset Diet recipes to include them.

Each day choose no more than two of the following:

- A Yellow Light seafood in place of Green Light seafood.
- Include an egg yolk in a recipe that used egg whites.
- Use dairy milk, up to the allowed quantities, in place of a non-dairy milk substitute.
- Add up to 1 ounce of cheese as a topping to a recipe that does not use it.

Keep in mind that some of these changes will add calories to the meal. If weight is a struggle for you and the diet was working as it was, you may need to make other adjustments to allow for the additional calories.

Remember that the goal is to not exceed a single high-iodine food per day or up to two medium-iodine foods per day. As an example, here are some typical adaptations you can make for the Maintenance phase. Note that these recipes all make multiple servings; the additional food item is meant to go into the complete recipe and be divided among the servings.

EGG YOLKS

1. Sweet Potato Hash (page 170): Use 2 eggs + ½ cup egg whites in place of 1 cup egg whites.
2. Three-Ingredient Pancakes (page 169): Use 2 whole eggs in place of ½ cup egg whites.
3. Vanilla Millet Hot Cereal (page 172): Reduce water by ½ cup; add 2 whole eggs to other ingredients.

DAIRY PRODUCTS

1. Mediterranean Fennel Salad (page 180): Add 3 ounces of chunked feta cheese and stir in before serving.
2. Thyroid Friendly Pesto (page 236): After blending, add 2 ounces grated parmesan cheese and blend for an additional 5 to 10 seconds.
3. Easy Breakfast Oatmeal (page 167): Substitute 2 ounces unsweetened Greek yogurt for non-dairy yogurt.

SEAFOOD

1. Garlic-Lime Calamari (page 224): Substitute yellowtail or salmon steaks for the calamari, increase the cooking time to 3 to 5 minutes for the first side and 2 to 3 minutes after turning. (This change counts as 1 high-iodine food per person.)
2. Chermoula Baked River Trout (page 225): Substitute salmon for river trout. (This change counts as 1 moderate-iodine food per person.)
3. One-Pot Green Chile Pasta (page 214): Add one 14.5-ounce can of baby clams, drained; include clams when adding the tomatoes and green chiles. (This change counts as 1 moderate-iodine food per person.)

RESTAURANT OPTIONS

As easy as it is to follow the Maintenance phase at home, you will want to eat out from time to time. When you do, it's best to be prepared. During the Reset phase, you focused on making food at home as much as possible. This was a time when your thyroid could have a chance to recover. The reality for most of us is that restaurant meals make up at least some of our food. There is a certain risk inherent in food you don't control, so do your best to minimize exposure. Thankfully, most restaurants' ability to adjust and meet special dietary needs is at an all-time high.

Here are some of your best options to stay true to the Thyroid Reset Diet guidelines while eating away from home.

BRING SALT

Salt is one of the hardest variables to control. A good strategy is to ask to have your food prepared without salt. Bring a small container of your own, and add to your food when it is served. Most outdoor sports and camping stores have salt containers made for backpacking. These often take up no more room in your purse or pocket than a small set of keys.

AVOID OBVIOUS INGREDIENTS

Stay away from dishes that are made primarily with high-iodine foods. Some straightforward ones to avoid would be seaweed salad, bread pudding, cream-based soups, breaded meats, and cheese pizza.

LOOK FOR HIDDEN IODINE

Sauces are often made with iodized salt, molasses, fish sauce, or other high-iodine ingredients. Stuffed meats like chicken breasts can often include bread crumbs. Grilled vegetables may be coated with butter.

Carry a card that says:

> Dear Chef,
>
> Due to a medical condition, I am on a regulated iodine diet. I must avoid foods with the smallest amounts of iodized salt, dairy products, seafood, sea vegetables, egg yolks, commercially baked bread products, and molasses.
>
> I have no restrictions on kosher salt, legumes, vegetables, fruits, egg whites, herbs, spices, vinegar, oil, nuts, seeds, meat, pork, or poultry.
>
> Thank you for your help!

Since many people monitor their dietary iodine before thyroid surgeries or procedures, chefs and cooks at busy restaurants have probably seen cards like this before and should be happy to accommodate you. The exception is fast-food stops and chain restaurants, which receive much of their food already processed.

SAFEST BETS

Take these guidelines into account when choosing your restaurant. Once you arrive, here are some ideas that are your likely best options:

Safer Ingredients

- Fresh meat and poultry
- Garlic
- Nut butter
- Oil and vinegar
- Pasta (not egg noodles)
- Tofu
- Tomato-based sauces
- Tomatillo sauces
- Vegetables

Best Main Dishes

- Baked chicken
- Grilled chicken
- Salads (hold the cheese, croutons, and dairy-based dressings)
- Steak
- Stir-fries

Best Side Dishes

- Baked potato
- Black beans
- Grilled vegetables
- Hummus
- Refried beans
- Rice paper spring rolls
- Steamed rice
- Steamed vegetables
- Stuffed grape leaves
- Tabbouleh

Best Breads (if made on site)

- Corn tortillas
- Naan
- Pita

Safest Desserts

- Baked fruit
- Date and nut butter balls
- Poached fruit
- Sorbets
- Stewed fruits

OTHER SOURCES OF IODINE

During the Maintenance phase, it is important to continue avoiding all supplements that contain iodine. It is also important to continue avoiding the use of cosmetics that may be high in iodine.

In future visits with doctors, be alert for iodine in medications or as a contract aid. If a doctor prescribes a new medication, double-check the medication list in Chapter Four. If your new medication is a high source of iodine, explain your situation to the prescriber and see if there is a substitute.

ADOPT A THYROID-FRIENDLY LIFESTYLE

Along with the right foods and pills, your daily habits can make or break your thyroid function. Take a closer look at your daily habits and make sure you're not compromising your health and your thyroid function. Here are some tips.

GET ENOUGH SLEEP

You likely know that sleep is a good idea in general. Sleep is also essential to keep your thyroid healthy. Here are a few things we've learned from recent studies:

- Lack of quality sleep for a single night can disrupt the thyroid-pituitary-hypothalamic axis.[5] These effects may be even worse in women.[6]
- Two nights of poor sleep can disrupt nearly all a healthy woman's hormones. Those shown to be affected include TSH, T3, T4, follicle-stimulating hormone (FSH), growth hormone, prolactin, estradiol, and luteinizing hormone (LH).[7]
- Too little sleep can be one of the largest drivers of autoimmune disease.[8] In fact, sleeping less than 7 hours per night has been shown to lead to the development of lupus.[9]
- Obstructive sleep apnea can lead to autoimmune thyroid disease.[10]
- Sleep disorders apart from apnea can lead to autoimmune thyroid disease.

You sleep well if most nights you can:

1. Quickly fall asleep without sleep aids, natural or prescription.
2. Don't wake your sleep partner by moving or snoring.
3. Sleep at least 7½ to 8 hours.
4. Wake up feeling rested without an alarm.
5. Don't fall asleep in the daytime when you intend to be awake.

If you have trouble sleeping, avoid conventional sleep aids like zolpidem (Ambien) or alprazolam (Xanax). Regular use of these or related medications has been shown to raise the risk of depression, cognitive impairment, certain cancers, and early death.[11] Shockingly, some studies have shown up to a fourfold increase in death rates with as few as 1 to 18 pills per year.[12]

If you don't fit the above criteria for sleeping well, work with your doctor immediately to find a reason. At Integrative Health, we do sleep studies on most of our patients with thyroid disease. There are now medically validated versions of these tests that you can do at home, with minimal disruption to your routines.

EXERCISE REGULARLY

What if there were a pill that was clinically proven to help people with thyroid disease, that would improve energy, lower anxiety, improve TSH and T3 levels, and heal the immune system? Exercise has been proven to do all of that and more.

In one study, people who had undergone complete removal of their thyroid glands owing to thyroid cancer were randomized into one of two groups. One group was just monitored; the other was trained in a simple exercise program that could be done at home. Those who were assigned to the exercise program did better in every measurable way.[13]

The exercises were very simple. Participants were advised to walk three days per week at 50 minutes per walk, or five days per week at 30 minutes per walk. Also, they did bodyweight strength training like push-ups and sit-ups twice weekly. Finally, they included 5 minutes of stretching before and after each exercise session. They put in 40 minutes per day for an average of five days per week on low- to moderate-intensity exercises.

I highly recommend a regular exercise regime to keep your thyroid healthy. If you don't have such a regime now, it's a perfect time to start. After your thyroid function has improved, there are some basic steps you can take to keep it from lapsing. These are worth sticking with over the long term!

FINDING THE RIGHT MEDICAL TEAM

A common theme expressed by those with thyroid disease is a sense of frustration with their initial healthcare providers. Often, symptoms go on for too long before thyroid disease is diagnosed. Even after diagnosis, treatments fail to alleviate many of the symptoms.

Sometimes the most important things are the hardest. Unraveling the symptoms of thyroid disease often does take an orchestrated effort between you and a doctor. You should never surrender your common sense and go along with approaches that seem unscientific or unsafe. You should also never ignore apparent side effects of treatments or abnormal blood levels just because a doctor says these are "healing crises" or that "it is okay to ignore the blood test."

Please know that your best recovery will come from having a healthy relationship with a professional. Ideally, it will be a person or a team of people who understand three things:

1. The power of diet to correct thyroid disease.
2. The importance of gently bringing your thyroid levels back to the optimal range for you.
3. How to identify and treat the other conditions that often exist alongside thyroid disease.

The best providers will be good communicators. You should feel that their top concern is not their pet theory or their income but, rather, your well-being. The best providers are those who connect with you and encourage you to settle for a level of health as good as, if not better than, you had before the thyroid diagnosis.

You can't meet with every potential thyroid doctor. Thankfully, there are some easy ways you can do prescreening to narrow down your list. Here are some of the most important considerations.

DO THEY FOCUS ON THYROID DISEASE?

Many functional doctors advertise that they treat thyroid disease, which is less of a draw when they also treat everything else.

To make this point, I just did a Google search for "local doctor thyroid disease." The top result also offers services related to mental health, autoimmunity, medical aesthetics, Type 2 diabetes, nutrition, weight loss, back pain, biohacking, ADHD, hormone replacement, leaky gut, and insomnia. Doctors have limits on their time, just as you do. To treat a condition well, it takes experience, activity in a community of peers, and ongoing training.

ARE THEY TRAINED IN LIFESTYLE MEDICINE?

The evidence is clear that diet, sleep, exercise, time in nature, social connections, and mind-set are among the most powerful parts of your recovery. Your thyroid doctor should also feel the same way and should be able to integrate it as a central part of your health care.

Doctors with training in lifestyle medicine may mention it directly, or they may have affiliation with groups such as the American Association of Naturopathic Physicians, American College of Lifestyle Medicine, or the American College of Preventive Medicine.

DO THEY OFFER TELEMEDICINE?

This consideration is not essential, but most people prefer it.

The telemedicine revolution has arrived. Many people may not happen to have the ideal thyroid doctor in their neighborhood. With telemedicine, you can work with doctors farther away or, in some cases, even out of state.

Thyroid care lends itself to telemedicine because it is focused on communicating your symptoms and progress, reviewing your lab findings, and making recommendations for changes in lifestyle, supplements, and medications. All these steps work fine from a distance. The newer telemedicine systems allow real-time, face-to-face communication with your doctor. You no longer must worry about traveling to and from a doctor's office or the wait times involved.

DO THEY TAKE INSURANCE?

This point may not be what you expect. If a doctor you are considering does take your insurance, he or she may have fewer options for you. Insurance companies have strict guidelines about the types of care a doctor can offer. More and more doctors are opting out of insurance and working directly with patients.

ARE THEY PART OF A TEAM?

There is nothing more frustrating than getting good momentum with a doctor and then not being able to find time to see him or her. Perhaps the doctor gets booked up too far in advance or maybe he is on vacation when you need him. Ideally, your doctor would be part of a team that shares the same training and approach to thyroid care. If your main doctor is not available, one of the others can step right in.

QUESTIONS TO FIND THE RIGHT TEAM

Once you have narrowed down your search, you may still have a few candidates to consider. Many doctors will offer a brief visit at which you can learn more about their approach. Those who have a more thorough online presence may also answer these questions on their website. The other option is that the doctor's team might be able to answer some of these questions as well.

One of the most important questions is: Do you think I can get better? Often doctors assume that thyroid disease cannot be improved. It can. You can feel as well as you did before it started. Never buy into lower expectations.

Here are some questions you should ask a potential choice of doctor. (If you'd like to bring this list with you to a medical visit, there is a printable version at www.thyroidresetdiet.com/resources.)

Do you ever use natural desiccated thyroid? The best doctors are willing to use any safe medication that can help you feel better. Natural desiccated thyroid medication contains T4, T3, T2, and thyroid proteins; it can help metabolism more than synthetic thyroid and can reverse autoimmunity.

Should I be screened for thyroid cancer? Thyroid cancer is the fastest-growing cancer type among women in North America. The best thyroid doctors screen all patients routinely and know how to adjust care if the patient has nodules, calcifications, or other risk factors.

When should I do my blood tests? If you have your blood taken at the wrong time of day, the results can be meaningless. The best doctors advise their patients on how to time their tests correctly and consider the time of day, fasting, thyroid medication, certain supplements, and the menstrual cycle. They also can suspect timing factors as a reason when blood levels are unusual.

What range is best on my blood tests? The best doctors understand the distinction between normal ranges and optimal levels. They also know how to personalize optimal levels for a given individual.

How would I know if I were taking too much medicine? The best thyroid doctors know that thyroid medicine can be dangerous when overdosed. Their goal is to help ease your symptoms, and they use blood tests to make sure they do so safely. For example, a prescription can be too high or an overdose can happen when your body recovers, as it did with Tasha (see below).

Case Story: Tasha

Tasha was a woman who attended my live events on Instagram and Facebook for years. She had Hashimoto's disease and struggled with fatigue and hair loss. She was kind and enthusiastic and I was always happy to see her name when I went live. Over time it became apparent to me that she was not improving much at all.

She knew enough and asked good questions, but she kept meeting roadblocks with her medical team. They were not willing to change her from T4-only medication and they did not see the merit in treating her anemia. I could not treat her over social media, and I encouraged her to connect with one of the doctors at Integrative Health or a local doctor who could help her further.

I thought of her as soon as telemedicine became available. My social media team reached out to her and explained how she now did not need to travel.

It turned out that Tasha had followed the guidelines in the Thyroid Reset Diet and her thyroid got better, but her prior doctors did not lower her medication. Within the first few months, her symptoms resolved. Education and self-care are essential, but you can make progress so much faster when you are not going at it alone.

ACTION STEPS TO TAKE NOW

- Is your next medical visit scheduled? Get it set up now even if it is a year out.
- Think through your lifestyle. What aspects of it are excellent? What parts of it can you improve this month?

The next chapter includes a comprehensive food list. In it, you will find nearly every food option categorized as Green Light, Yellow Light, or Red Light. Prepare to be amazed at how many Green Light options you will find!

Chapter Seven

Food Lists and Meal Assembly

Here, you'll find a complete list of foods from which to choose, along with ideas on assembling your meals if following a meal plan doesn't work for your dietary habits.

The food lists are organized by category, whether Green Light, Yellow Light, or Red Light, based on its iodine content. The meal assembly gives you some general ideas on constructing your meals using thyroid-friendly dishes.

THE FOOD LISTS

The goal during the Reset phase is to stay on Green Light foods and avoid Yellow Light and Red Light foods. During the Maintenance phase, you are welcome to add up to two foods from the Yellow Light food list each day. You can still freely eat Green Light foods, but you should continue to avoid Red Light foods.

SERVING SIZES

For some of the food items, I specify serving sizes, and for others I do not. Some foods have consistent amounts of iodine, so maintaining the stated serving size is important. Many other foods contain so little iodine, however, that the serving size does not matter—you won't get too much iodine even if you eat a lot of them. Finally, some foods have so much iodine that it will be too much for you even in the smallest practical serving size.

BEVERAGES

Water

Purified drinking water is not a significant source of iodine. There are some parts of the world in which untreated water has significant amounts, but this is not the norm.

Alcohol

Substantial evidence suggests that alcohol can be harmful to thyroid function.[1] Therefore, it is best to avoid alcohol during the Reset phase. However, in the Maintenance phase, a few servings of wine or beer per week likely have no significant effect on thyroid function. Please know that evidence no longer supports the claim that wine is a healthy option. If you have small amounts on occasion, the harm is likely negligible, but don't think you are missing out on some benefits if you avoid it.

Green Light Beverages

- Coffee, all types, with no dairy, no flavorings
- Mineral water, sparkling water
- Tea, all types, with no dairy, no flavorings

Yellow Light Beverages

- Alcoholic beverages: wine, beer

Red Light Beverages

- Dairy-based protein powder, whey, casein, dry milk
- Flavored coffees
- Hard liquor
- Meal replacement beverages without a stated iodine content

CONDIMENTS

Many condiments are highly concentrated foods and should be used in appropriately small proportions for a healthy diet. Even if they are safe for your thyroid, your health may be otherwise compromised if you eat too much of them.

Note that many of the recipes use an oil mister; this is quite helpful to have, as it allows you to fill the canister with your desired oil (I prefer avocado oil) and then apply a light mist of the oil to a baking pan or skillet, thereby limiting the amount of oil you need to cook an item.

Green Light Condiments

- All cooking oils; preferred options include avocado, canola, olive
- Earth Balance and Smart Balance spreads
- Guacamole
- Herbs and spices (full list on page 135)
- Hummus
- Ketchup
- Marinara sauce
- Mustard
- Salsa
- Sweeteners: honey, lo han, maple syrup, stevia, xylitol
- Tamari, coconut aminos
- Vegan mayonnaise
- Vinegar, all types

Yellow Light Condiments

- Aioli, up to 2 tablespoons
- Brown sugar, up to 2 teaspoons
- Fish sauce, up to 2 teaspoons
- Mayonnaise, up to 2 tablespoons
- Pesto, up to 2 tablespoons
- Sucanat, up to 2 teaspoons
- Tartar sauce, up to 2 teaspoons
- Turbinado sugar, up to 2 teaspoons
- Worcestershire sauce, up to 2 teaspoons

Red Light Condiments

- Duck sauce
- Hoisin sauce
- Molasses
- Sweet and sour sauce
- Teriyaki sauce
- Tzatziki
- Whipped cream

DAIRY PRODUCTS

This category includes all foods made from the milk of a mammal, whether a cow, camel, goat, or sheep.

Green Light Dairy

- Non-dairy substitutes for milk, cheese, butter, yogurt, cheese, and ice cream are safe. Be sure they are free of seaweed extracts such as carrageenan. They can be made from almond, soy, flax, coconut, oat, hemp, or other vegan sources.

If you would like a comprehensive list of dairy substitutes checked for safety on the Thyroid Reset Diet, visit www.thyroidresetdiet.com/resources.

Yellow Light Dairy

- Butter (ghee, or clarified butter), up to 2 teaspoons
- Cheese (any type), up to 1 ounce
- Gelato or ice cream (all types), up to ¼ cup
- Mayonnaise, up to 1 tablespoon
- Milk (any type), up to ¼ cup
- Sour cream, up to 1 tablespoon
- Yogurt (any type), up to 2 ounces by weight

Red Light Dairy

- All other dairy products from milk from cows, goats, or sheep
- Any Yellow Light foods in amounts above recommended

EGGS

Eggs are substantial sources of iodine, but iodine is found only in the yolks; egg whites are iodine-free. Two egg whites can replace a whole egg in most recipes. Note that some vegan egg products contain carrageenan and should be avoided.

Green Light Eggs

- Egg-free products: Aquafaba, Bob's Red Mill Egg Replacer, Just Egg Plant-Based, The Neat Egg substitute, Egg Replacer
- Egg products: Egg Beaters, egg whites, egg white protein powder

Yellow Light Eggs

- Egg yolk, up to 1

Red Light Eggs

- Agar-agar as an egg replacement
- Baked goods with whole eggs
- Dried eggs
- Egg noodles
- Egg yolks (over 1)
- Hollandaise sauce
- Powdered eggs
- Whole eggs

FRUITS

Fruits are a food category that is almost universally safe. However, cantaloupe that has been commercially cubed and frozen is unusually high in iodine. Other outliers are prunes and prune juice. With these exceptions, fresh, frozen, dried, and unsalted canned fruit are all safe options.

Green Light Fruits

- Apples
- Apricots
- Avocados
- Bananas
- Blood oranges
- Blueberries
- Cranberries
- Dates
- Figs
- Grapefruit
- Grapes
- Kiwi
- Lemons
- Mandarin oranges
- Mangoes
- Navel oranges
- Papaya
- Pears
- Peaches
- Pineapple
- Plums
- Raisins
- Strawberries
- Valencia oranges
- Watermelon

Yellow Light Fruits

- Canned fruit with salt or sugar
- Commercially prepared frozen cantaloupe

- Frozen fruit with salt or sugar
- Prune juice, up to ½ cup
- Prunes, up to 1 ounce

Red Light Fruits

- Sea buckthorn

FERMENTED FOODS

Sauerkraut and most other fermented vegetables are generally safe because it is thought that iodine could disrupt the fermentation process. Summer Bock, a fermentationist, stated that the typical recommendations for fermented vegetables encourage iodine-free salt out of concern for the disruption of beneficial bacterial development from the antimicrobial properties of iodized salt. Kimchi may be the one exception; commercial versions of kimchi are often high in iodine because it is traditionally made with shrimp and fish extracts.[2]

Green Light Foods

- Kombucha
- Miso
- Natto
- Sauerkraut
- Soy sauce
- Tempeh

Yellow Light Foods

- Buttermilk, up to ¼ cup
- Kefir, up to ¼ cup
- Kimchi, up to 1 ounce
- Yogurt, up to 2 ounces by weight

Red Light Foods

- None

GRAIN PRODUCTS

Whole grains contain no significant amount of iodine. They are Green Light foods regardless of serving size; these also include whole-grain flours. But there is an important nuance with grains. Commercially baked products are Red Light foods because they are often made with iodine-based ingredients that are not part of home baking recipes.

Green Light Grains

- All intact whole grains and grain flours for home use with no added salt
- Amaranth
- Barley
- Buckwheat groats
- Buckwheat noodles
- Bulgur
- Corn
- Einkorn
- Farro
- Freekeh (unripe bulgur)
- Kamut
- Matzo bread and matzo meal
- Millet
- Oats and oatmeal
- Pasta, with no added salt
- Popcorn
- Quinoa
- Rice and unsalted rice cakes
- Sorghum
- Spelt
- Teff
- Triticale
- Udon noodles
- Wheat berries
- Wild rice

Yellow Light Grains

- None

Red Light Grains

- Bagels
- Baking mixes
- Breads
- Cereals
- Cookies
- Cornbread

- Crackers
- Croissants
- Gluten-free bread
- Microwave popcorn
- Muffins
- Pancakes
- Tortillas

HERBS AND SPICES

All herbs and spices (without added salt) are allowed.

Green Light Herbs and Spices

- Ajwain
- Allspice
- Anise
- Annatto
- Arrowroot
- Asafetida
- Basil
- Bay leaves
- Black pepper
- Cacao
- Caraway
- Cardamom
- Celery seeds
- Chervil
- Chiles
- Chives
- Cilantro
- Cinnamon
- Citrus zest
- Cloves
- Coriander
- Cumin
- Curry leaves
- Dill
- Fennel
- Fenugreek
- Garlic
- Lemongrass
- Long pepper
- Mace
- Mustard
- Nutmeg
- Oregano
- Paprika
- Parsley
- Poppy seeds
- Rosemary
- Saffron
- Sage
- Star anise
- Sumac
- Summer savory
- Tarragon
- Thyme
- Turmeric
- Vanilla extract
- Wasabi
- White pepper

Yellow Light Herbs and Spices

- None

Red Light Herbs and Spices

- Herbs and spices in Red Light foods or highly processed foods, such as the basil in pesto with cheese

LEGUMES

Legumes do not contain significant amounts of iodine. For commercially canned beans, choose versions without added salt or flavorings.

Green Light Legumes

- All dried beans and legumes
- Adzuki beans
- Broad beans
- Cannellini beans
- Chickpeas
- Cowpeas
- Great northern beans
- Green beans
- Kidney beans
- Lentils
- Lima beans
- Natto
- Navy beans
- Peas
- Pinto beans
- Soybeans
- Soy protein powder
- Tempeh
- Tigernuts
- Tofu
- White beans

Yellow Light Legumes

- Canned beans with salt, up to ½ cup
- Canned green beans with salt, up to ½ cup
- Frozen beans with salt, up to ½ cup
- Refried beans, up to ½ cup (unless homemade with iodine-free salt)

Red Light Legumes

- None

MEATS AND POULTRY

Meats and poultry contain some iodine, but the amounts are consistent and not significant at the quantities typically eaten. All unprocessed and unseasoned meat and poultry are in the Green Light category. Cured and processed meats are all unsafe, owing to their iodine content.

Green Light Meats and Poultry

- Beef or calves liver
- Beef roast
- Beef steak
- Chicken, white or dark meat
- Chicken livers
- Ground beef
- Ground chicken
- Ground lamb
- Ground pork
- Ground turkey
- Lamb roast
- Kidneys
- Pork chops
- Pork roast
- Pork tenderloin
- Quail
- Rabbit
- Turkey, white or dark meat
- Venison

Yellow Light Meats and Poultry

- None

Red Light Meats and Poultry

- Bacon
- Bologna
- Bratwurst
- Braunschweiger
- Corned beef
- Ham
- Kielbasa
- Pepperoni
- Salami
- Sausage

NUTS AND SEEDS

Like other plant foods, nuts and seeds are safe, as are lightly toasted nuts and seeds or nut and seed butters. Only the versions that have added salt are important to avoid. Raw nuts and seeds can be roasted at home and salted with non-iodized salt.

Green Light Nuts and Seeds

- Almond butter
- Almonds
- Brazil nuts
- Cashew butter
- Cashews
- Chestnuts
- Chia seeds
- Coconut
- Filberts
- Flaxseed
- Hemp seeds
- Macadamia nuts
- Peanut butter, natural
- Peanuts
- Pecans
- Pine nuts
- Pistachios
- Pumpkin seeds
- Sesame seeds
- Sunflower butter
- Sunflower seeds
- Tahini
- Walnuts

Yellow Light Nuts and Seeds

- Commercially roasted nuts and seeds
- Nuts and seeds with seasonings or flavorings

Red Light Nuts and Seeds

- None

SALT

What about all the processed foods with added salt? Of course, you're better off with less processed food in your diet. It turns out that most processed food from packages or restaurants is made without iodized salt. An odd exception is Burger King.[3] In general, you will do well if you keep processed foods to a rarity and avoid the other main sources of invisible iodine.

Green Light Salts

- Canning or pickling salt
- Celtic brand sea salt, light gray, coarse or fine
- Kosher salt
- Table salt, non-iodized

Yellow Light Salts

- None

Red Light Salts

- Himalayan salt
- Iodized salt
- Sea salts
- Unspecified salt

FISH AND SEAFOOD

Since all iodine comes from the sea, seafood is a significant source of iodine. Freshwater fish, however, is low in iodine and many of its types are safe to use. Also, the amount of iodine found in seafood can vary tremendously from type to type. Even some types of seafood have inconsistent levels of iodine and a few types have consistently low levels. Because of the clear health benefits of seafood, I worked hard to include some in the diet.

Green Light Fish and Seafood

Some of these fish can be found from salt water or fresh water. Be sure they are from fresh water. If they are from salt water, they will likely be too high in iodine.

- Anchovies, up to ½ ounce
- Bass, fresh water, lake or river, up to 4 ounces

- Carp, up to 4 ounces
- Catfish, up to 4 ounces
- Crappie, up to 4 ounces
- Octopus, up to 4 ounces
- Perch, river, up to 4 ounces
- Scallops, up to 4 ounces
- Shrimp, without shell, and boiled, up to 4 ounces
- Squid, up to 4 ounces
- Tilapia, up to 4 ounces
- Trout, rainbow or river, up to 4 ounces
- Walleye, fresh water, up to 4 ounces

Yellow Light Fish and Seafood

- Clams, shucked, up to 4 ounces short-necked
- Flounder, up to 4 ounces
- Mackerel, up to 4 ounces
- Ocean perch, up to 4 ounces
- River trout, up to 4 ounces
- Salmon, up to 4 ounces
- Sardines, up to 4 ounces
- Shrimp, with shell and/or not boiled, up to 4 ounces
- Snow crab, up to 4 ounces
- Tuna, albacore, canned in water
- Tuna, chunk light, canned in water
- Yellowtail tuna, up to 4 ounces

Red Light Fish and Seafood

- Abalone
- Anglerfish
- Blue crab
- Clams, canned
- Cod
- Haddock
- Lobster
- Ocean walleye
- Oysters
- Pacific cod
- Pollock
- Swordfish

SEA VEGETABLES

Sea vegetables have the highest levels of iodine and no safe options. Spirulina or chlorella can be used, but only in the Maintenance phase and not above the recommended serving size.

Green Light Sea Vegetables

- None

Yellow Light Sea Vegetables

- Chlorella, up to 3 grams
- Spirulina, up to 3 grams

Red Light Sea Vegetables

- Agar-agar[4]
- Alaria
- Arame
- Bladderwrack
- Dulse
- Hijiki
- Kelp
- Kombu
- Laminaria (nori)
- Sea buckthorn (technically a fruit)
- Wakame

VEGETABLES

Fresh vegetables do not contain significant amounts of iodine. Once you exclude vegetables that are canned or frozen with added salt, vegetables of all types are safe to include. Not only are they safe, but the Thyroid Reset Diet also advocates a minimum of five servings per day. Consider 1 cup as a serving.

Green Light Vegetables

- Asparagus, fresh or frozen
- Beets, fresh or canned
- Bell pepper

- Black olives
- Broccoli, fresh or frozen
- Cabbage, fresh
- Carrots, baby or full size
- Cauliflower, fresh or frozen
- Celery
- Chicory
- Chinese cabbage
- Chives
- Collards, fresh or frozen
- Cucumber
- Daikon
- Delicata squash
- Edamame
- Eggplant
- Ginger, fresh
- Green pepper
- Horseradish
- Jackfruit
- Jerusalem artichoke
- Lettuce, iceberg or leaf
- Mushrooms, button, maitake, oyster shiitake
- Mustard greens
- Okra fresh or frozen
- Onion
- Parsley
- Peas, sugar snap or English
- Potatoes, peeled
- Pumpkin
- Shallot
- Spinach, fresh or frozen
- Squash, winter, fresh or frozen
- Summer squash or zucchini
- Sweet potatoes
- Tomatoes
- Turnip greens and root

Yellow Light Vegetables

- Mixed vegetables, frozen with salt, up to 1 cup
- Potatoes, with peel, up to 1 cup

Red Light Vegetables

- Vegetables packed or seasoned with Red Light seasonings

MEAL ASSEMBLY

Now that you have lists of safe foods to use, what are the best ways to combine these ingredients into meals? In earlier chapters, I emphasized the importance of protein, lots of fresh produce, the right amounts of fats, and some carbs as the basis for your meals. The easiest way to get this combination is to think about your meals in terms of protein, produce, and carbs, with an optional sprinkling of fats. Fats are not essential at every meal; in fact, our human requirement for essential fats is easy to meet.

In our home, we usually try one to two new recipes each week, but most of the time we do more of a meal-assembly process. We first take an inventory of what we have on hand that is perishable. Usually the protein and produce have the shortest refrigerator life. We also see if we have any carbs that have been cooked already, like some leftover rice or potatoes. From there, we decide what flavors we're in the mood for and we add the seasonings.

When assembling your meals, always be sure to check the food lists and consider the ingredients.

MEAL ASSEMBLY IDEAS FOR BREAKFAST

The most popular healthy breakfasts are shakes, hot cereals, and skillet dishes. Of these, shakes are my favorite. They take the least time and are the easiest way to pack in the most nutrients to start the day. Chapter Eight has many versions if you'd like to try some new flavors. Here are the fundamentals.

Protein Shake Basic Recipe

SERVES 1

With shakes, separate carbs are often not needed, since the shakes include fruit and/or beans. This is the basic recipe, which you can adapt to suit whatever ingredients you have available.

PROTEIN

- Liquid egg whites, 1 cup
- Soft tofu, 4 ounces
- Vegetable-based protein powder, 1 serving as per package

PRODUCE

- Banana, 1 medium, peeled
- Berries, fresh or frozen, ½ cup
- Mango, frozen, cubed, ½ cup
- White beans and liquid, ½ cup

FLAVORINGS

- Almond extract, ½ teaspoon
- Chia seeds, 1 to 2 tablespoons
- Ground cinnamon, to taste
- Stevia, to taste
- Sunflower seeds, 1 to 2 tablespoons
- Vanilla extract, ½ teaspoon

In a high-speed blender, combine the protein, produce, and flavorings with 1 cup water and 1 cup ice and blend for 1 to 2 minutes, or until smooth. Non-dairy milk can be used in place of the water to thicken the texture and boost the flavor. I usually prefer canned beans instead, like navy, great northern, or cannellini; they add taste and texture, and offer more nutrition. If using canned beans, also add the canning liquid for best results. If you're looking for a crunchy texture, add nuts or fruit after the initial blending, then blend for a final 5 to 10 seconds.

Hot Cereal Basic Recipe

SERVES 1

I usually enjoy hot cereal with a protein drink on the side. Since the hot cereal is nearly a meal unto itself, I use a flavored protein powder (with no added sugar), mixed with just water and ice. You can also add one of the protein options for the Protein Shake (page 144) in the final stages of cooking; be sure to mix constantly while simmering for 3 minutes.

CARBS (CHOOSE 1 OPTION)

- Buckwheat groats, ¼ cup
- Leftover cooked brown rice, ¾ cup
- Old-fashioned rolled oats, ½ cup
- Steel-cut oats, ¼ cup

PRODUCE (CHOOSE 1 OR 2 OPTIONS)

- Apple, ½ medium, diced
- Banana, ½ medium, peeled and sliced
- Pear, ½ medium, diced
- Raisins, ¼ cup

FLAVORINGS (AS DESIRED)

- Almond extract, ½ teaspoon
- Chia seeds, 1 to 2 tablespoons
- Coconut flakes, 1 tablespoon
- Ground cardamom, to taste
- Ground cinnamon, to taste
- Stevia, to taste
- Vanilla extract, ½ teaspoon
- Walnuts, chopped, ¼ cup

In a medium saucepan, measure out the carb and add 2 to 3 parts water per 1 part carb, based on how thick you like your cereal. Add the remaining ingredients and stir well. Bring to a low simmer, then cover and simmer for 15 minutes. Let rest for 10 minutes, still covered, before eating.

NOTE: It works well to cook several servings in advance and store them in the refrigerator.

Skillet Dish Basic Recipe

SERVES 1

These are the familiar breakfast skillets, usually based on eggs and potatoes. They are flexible and can work well with a big variety of ingredients and seasonings. I do include lean versions of cured meat. High amounts of cured meat can be harmful, but if you average under an ounce per day, and include legumes and vegetables, there is no evidence of harm.

PROTEIN (CHOOSE 1 OR ½ OF 2 OPTIONS)

- Canadian bacon, 2 slices
- Cooked poultry or beef, ½ cup
- Extra-firm tofu, diced, 4 ounces
- Liquid egg whites, 1 cup
- Tempeh, diced, 4 ounces

CARBS (CHOOSE 1 OR ½ OF 2 OPTIONS)

- Black beans, ½ cup
- Pinto beans, ½ cup
- Plantain, diced, ½ cup
- Potato, 1 medium, diced
- Sweet potato, diced, ½ cup

PRODUCE (UNLIMITED)

- Cauliflower, diced
- Onion, diced
- Spinach leaves
- Tomatoes, diced
- Zucchini, diced

FLAVORINGS (AS DESIRED)

- Chili powder
- Chives, chopped
- Garlic, fresh or dried
- Green chiles, canned
- Non-dairy plain yogurt, 1 to 2 tablespoons (add after cooking in place of sour cream)
- Oregano, dried or fresh, to taste
- Salsa
- Salt and pepper

In a medium skillet, sauté the onions, garlic, and spices. Remove them, then sauté any vegetables until tender. Remove them, and cook or reheat the protein. Combine all the ingredients and add the seasonings.

NOTE: When cooking potatoes, I prefer to use leftover boiled or baked potatoes; if these are not available, I microwave a potato for 3 to 4 minutes, let it cool for a few minutes, and then dice it into the skillet. Otherwise, diced raw potatoes need at least 10 minutes of sautéing until done.

MEAL ASSEMBLY IDEAS FOR LUNCH AND DINNER

Easy lunches and dinners include salads, stir-fries, soups, and wraps.

Salad Basic Recipe

SERVES 1

PROTEIN (CHOOSE 1 OPTION)

- Chicken breast, cooked and diced, ½ cup
- Dried seasoned tofu, diced, ½ cup
- Lean stew meat, cooked and diced, ½ cup

PRODUCE (UNLIMITED)

- Broccoli florets
- Cucumber, diced
- Green onions, diced
- Greens, red-leaf, romaine, butter lettuce, spinach
- Mung bean sprouts
- Onion, diced
- Tomato, diced

CARBS (CHOOSE 1 OPTION)

- Cooked brown rice, ¾ cup
- Garbanzo beans, ½ cup

SEASONINGS (UNLIMITED EXCEPT AS NOTED)

- Anchovies, mashed, 1 tablespoon
- Apple cider vinegar
- Avocado, diced, ½ cup
- Chives, diced
- Extra-virgin olive oil
- Garlic, fresh or powdered
- Olives, sliced, ¼ cup
- Salt and pepper
- Tarragon, fresh or dried

Combine all the ingredients in a large bowl and mix well. Cover and refrigerate if preparing in advance. Stir in the seasonings just before serving. The best protein options are diced leftover protein from the evening before.

Soup Basic Recipe

SERVES 1

Perhaps more than any other dish, soups can be the repository for nearly any leftovers you have on hand. Find a stock or bouillon that you like. We like to make our own broths and freeze them.

PROTEIN (CHOOSE 1 OPTION)

- Chicken breast, cooked and diced, ½ cup
- Dried seasoned tofu, diced, ½ cup
- Lean stew meat, cooked and diced, ½ cup
- Tempeh, diced, ½ cup

PRODUCE (AT LEAST 2 CUPS TOTAL PER SERVING)

- Cabbage, finely sliced
- Carrots, sliced
- Celery, sliced
- Onions, diced
- Spinach, torn
- Zucchini, sliced

CARBS (½ TO ¾ CUP)

- Barley, pearled, cooked
- Brown rice, cooked
- Cannellini beans, canned
- Corn, frozen
- Lentils, cooked

LIQUID (UP TO 2 CUPS)

- Broth, stock, or bouillon powder
- Diced tomatoes, 15-ounce can

SEASONINGS (AS DESIRED)

- Garlic, ½ clove
- Ginger, fresh, grated, 1 teaspoon
- Lemongrass, ½ teaspoon
- Turmeric, ¼ teaspoon

For most soups, first sauté your onions, garlic, and seasonings, then set aside. Add your main vegetables and gently sauté, then set aside. Add your protein and sauté briefly. Add the previously sautéed ingredients, pour in the liquid—stock or water—and simmer until heated through.

Now you have a good sense of how to improvise in the kitchen. For those who need a little more structure, you'll find recipes and meal plans in the next chapter.

Chapter Eight

Recipes and Menu Plans

Now that you understand which foods are best for your thyroid, let's make your meals tasty and easy! These are recipes that Kirin, my wife, and I make regularly. I hope you enjoy them; my family and I love them all.

This chapter contains recipes that you can use in both the Reset and the Maintenance phases. Nearly every recipe has options for those who are AIP or vegan. Most recipes have a shortlist of ingredients you can find in any supermarket; a few have some more exotic ingredients in case you'd like to try something new. None of the recipes will take more than a few minutes to prepare.

Please know that you don't have to use just these recipes. It is easy to assemble meals that fit the Thyroid Reset Diet guidelines. You can always look at the food lists in Chapter Seven and swap ingredients as you see fit. You're also welcome to mix and match the recipes. Breakfast can be as simple as a shake. Lunch and dinner can be a batch-cooked protein, some basic greens, and some cooked grains or beans. You can also make a double-size shake for breakfast and keep half of it for a lunch on the go. Dinner recipes can be doubled, and the extra can serve as lunch the following day.

Many of the recipes are stand-alone meals. For those that are not, be sure to always have some mixture of protein, vegetables, and good carbs. The serving suggestions, provided when appropriate, help you out there.

If you are gluten-free, vegan, or AIP, you'll have lots of recipes to choose from. Many will work for you as they are. Most of the rest can be modified simply.

If you are new to cooking with whole grains and beans, you'll find cooking instructions, tips, and ways to help with digestibility at www.thyroidresetdiet.com/resources.

THE 28-DAY MEAL PLAN

If you'd like an idea of how to put these recipes together for your Reset phase, the following is a suggested meal plan.

		WEEK 1	PAGE
MONDAY	BREAKFAST	Chocolate Cherry Swirl	159
	LUNCH	Freekeh Tabbouleh	179
	DINNER	Sweet Corn and Sorghum Soup	194
TUESDAY	BREAKFAST	Easy Breakfast Oatmeal	167
	LUNCH	Mediterranean Fennel Salad	180
	DINNER	Dr. Khoshaba's Lentil Soup	195
WEDNESDAY	BREAKFAST	Chocolate Mint Shake	160
	LUNCH	Classic Niçoise Salad	181
	DINNER	Gingered Tempeh and Broccoli Basic Brown Rice	212 228
THURSDAY	BREAKFAST	Three-Ingredient Pancakes	169
	LUNCH	Chai Potato Bowl	184
	DINNER	15-Bean Soup	198
FRIDAY	BREAKFAST	Eggnog for Breakfast	161
	LUNCH	Healthy Caesar Salad	182
	DINNER	Calamari Stew	202
SATURDAY	BREAKFAST	Sweet Potato Hash	170
	LUNCH	Cilantro Shrimp Bowl	186
	DINNER	Kirin's Slow-Cooker Chicken Basic Greens Basic Brown Rice	213 229 228
SUNDAY	BREAKFAST	Ginger Spice Shake	162
	LUNCH	Roman Wrap	189
	DINNER	Homestyle Meatloaf Whole-Grain Sourdough Bread Basic Greens	203 232 229

		WEEK 2	PAGE
MONDAY	BREAKFAST	Peppermint Nut Butter Shake	163
	LUNCH	Classic Niçoise Salad	181
	DINNER	One-Pot Green Chile Pasta	214
TUESDAY	BREAKFAST	Huevos Rancheros	173
	LUNCH	Masala Lentil Wrap	190
	DINNER	Chicken with Peaches and Black Beans	216
WEDNESDAY	BREAKFAST	Pumpkin Pie Delight	164
	LUNCH	Mediterranean Fennel Salad	180
	DINNER	Creamy Lentil Curry	217
THURSDAY	BREAKFAST	Vanilla Millet Hot Cereal	172
	LUNCH	Sesame Ginger Lettuce Wrap	192
	DINNER	Shepherd's Pie	205
FRIDAY	BREAKFAST	Orange Spice Shake	165
	LUNCH	Southwest Scramble Wrap	193
	DINNER	Poached Garlic Chicken	219
SATURDAY	BREAKFAST	Huevos Rancheros	173
	LUNCH	Cilantro Shrimp Bowl	186
	DINNER	White Bean Chile Verde	196
SUNDAY	BREAKFAST	Apple Pie Shake	166
	LUNCH	Freekeh Tabbouleh	179
	DINNER	Homestyle Beef Stew	197

		WEEK 3	PAGE
MONDAY	BREAKFAST	Easy Breakfast Oatmeal	167
	LUNCH	Shiitake Soba Bowl	188
	DINNER	Minnesota-Style Wild Rice Hot Dish	207
TUESDAY	BREAKFAST	Three-Ingredient Pancakes	169
	LUNCH	Roman Wrap	189
	DINNER	Curried Kabocha Soup	201
WEDNESDAY	BREAKFAST	Sweet Potato Hash	170
	LUNCH	Healthy Caesar Salad	182
	DINNER	One-Pot Green Chile Pasta	214
THURSDAY	BREAKFAST	Apple Pie Shake	166
	LUNCH	Classic Niçoise Salad	181
	DINNER	Chermoula Baked River Trout	225
FRIDAY	BREAKFAST	Buckwheat Berry Porridge	171
	LUNCH	Sesame Ginger Lettuce Wrap	192
	DINNER	Better Than Carry-Out Orange Chicken	220
SATURDAY	BREAKFAST	Ginger Spice Shake	162
	LUNCH	Mediterranean Fennel Salad	180
	DINNER	Thyroid Friendly Pesto	236
SUNDAY	BREAKFAST	Vanilla Millet Hot Cereal	172
	LUNCH	Southwest Scramble Wrap	193
	DINNER	Cajun Catfish	222

		WEEK 4	PAGE
MONDAY	BREAKFAST	Overnight Apple Pie Oats	177
	LUNCH	Masala Lentil Wrap	190
	DINNER	Classic Split Pea Soup	200
TUESDAY	BREAKFAST	Whole Oat Porridge	175
	LUNCH	Roman Wrap	189
	DINNER	Creamy Tarragon Chicken	210
WEDNESDAY	BREAKFAST	Brazil Nut Quickbread	176
	LUNCH	Chai Potato Bowl	184
	DINNER	Chermoula Baked River Trout	225
THURSDAY	BREAKFAST	Buckwheat Banana Bread	178
	LUNCH	Shiitake Soba Bowl	188
	DINNER	Gingered Tempeh and Broccoli	212
FRIDAY	BREAKFAST	Pumpkin Pie Delight	164
	LUNCH	Cilantro Shrimp Bowl	186
	DINNER	Soup of the Green Goddess	199
SATURDAY	BREAKFAST	Huevos Rancheros	173
	LUNCH	Chai Potato Bowl	184
	DINNER	Kirin's Slow-Cooker Chicken	213
SUNDAY	BREAKFAST	Eggnog for Breakfast	161
	LUNCH	Classic Niçoise Salad	181
	DINNER	Paprika Chicken with Roasted Limas and Brussel Sprouts	209

WEEKLY SHOPPING LIST

You can see the weekly shopping lists for the 28-Day Meal Plan beginning on page 258 or obtain a printable download of them at www.thyroidresetdiet.com/resources.

BREAKFAST IDEAS

Your first meal can set the tone for the entire rest of the day. Yet typical breakfast foods like milk, eggs, and baked goods can push you into unsafe levels of iodine.

I do encourage you to eat breakfast. People who eat breakfast have an easier time retaining muscle mass, being less hungry in the evening, and regulating their cortisol levels. We also know that optimal protein can be important for thyroid function, and it can be hard to get without a solid breakfast. If you feel that avoiding breakfast has been helpful, please do your best to make up the nutrients in your other meals.

SHAKES

Shakes are one of the easiest ways to get the protein and fibers your body needs in the morning without your making an elaborate meal. Here are several of my favorite recipes, all adapted to fit the Thyroid Reset Diet.

- **PROTEIN POWDER OPTIONS** Since iodine is the largest concern with thyroid function, it is best to use protein powders that come from normally low-iodine foods and that are tested for their iodine content. Whey- and egg-based protein powders do run the risk of having high levels of iodine. Look out for those without added iodine, kelp, sea vegetables, or iodine texturizers like carrageenan. Even some of the vegetable protein raw materials that we have tested have had too much iodine to be safe. Pea or hemp proteins are often good options, but they should be assayed to show their iodine content. Our clinic uses the premade meal replacement Daily Reset Shake, which has been shown to have under 0.15 mcg of iodine per gram. You can visit www.thyroidresetdiet.com/resources for more detailed information.

- **BEANS IN SHAKES?** In the early 2000s, studies started coming out in droves about the health benefits of a food constituent called resistant starch. It was able to help people lose weight, lower blood sugar, and improve digestive health. I started to include beans in my shakes many years ago to add some more resistant starch. But the great taste and texture the beans add have made them indispensable. If ever I make a shake and don't have some beans to pour into it, I find it is nowhere near as creamy. My favorite trick is to use canned white beans or navy beans. I open the can and just pour in roughly one-third of a cup of beans along with the aquafaba (the canning liquid).

Chocolate Cherry Swirl

SERVES 1 **PREP TIME: 5 MINUTES** **TOTAL TIME: 5 MINUTES**

- 2 cups water or unflavored non-dairy milk
- 1 serving vanilla or unflavored vegetable-based protein powder
- 1 tablespoon unsweetened cocoa powder, natural or Dutch-process
- 1 to 2 Brazil nuts
- ½ cup packed fresh spinach
- 10 frozen cherries
- ½ frozen banana
- ½ cup crushed ice

In a high-speed blender, combine the water, protein powder, cocoa powder, Brazil nuts, spinach, cherries, and banana. Add the ice. Blend all the ingredients until smooth.

Chocolate Mint Shake

SERVES 1 **PREP TIME: 5 MINUTES** **TOTAL TIME: 5 MINUTES**

- 2 cups water or unflavored non-dairy milk
- 1 serving vanilla or unflavored vegetable-based protein powder
- 1 tablespoon unsweetened cocoa powder, natural or Dutch-process
- 1 to 2 Brazil nuts
- ½ cup packed fresh spinach
- ⅓ cup canned navy beans, with canning liquid
- 4 fresh mint leaves, or 2 drops peppermint extract
- ½ cup crushed ice

In a high-speed blender, combine the water, protein powder, cocoa powder, Brazil nuts, spinach, beans, and mint. Add the ice. Blend all the ingredients until smooth.

Eggnog for Breakfast

I loved eggnog as a kid. I've come to realize that it's more about the taste and texture than it is about the ingredients. This is a version that can turn eggnog into a year-round favorite.

SERVES 1   PREP TIME: **5 MINUTES**   TOTAL TIME: **5 MINUTES**

- 1 cup unsweetened flax milk or other non-dairy milk
- 1 serving vanilla or unflavored vegetable-based protein powder
- ¼ teaspoon freshly grated nutmeg
- ¼ teaspoon ground allspice
- ½ teaspoon vanilla extract
- 2 Medjool dates, pitted
- 2 teaspoons chopped raw cashews
- ⅓ cup canned navy beans, with canning liquid
- ½ cup crushed ice

In a high-powered blender, combine the flax milk, protein powder, nutmeg, allspice, vanilla, dates, cashews, and beans. Add the ice. Blend all the ingredients until smooth.

GLUTEN-FREE OPTION: No modification needed
VEGAN OPTION: No modification needed
AIP OPTION: Use AIP-approved protein source; use coconut yogurt instead of beans

Ginger Spice Shake

Entire books have been written about the health benefits of ginger. I like to store fresh ginger in the freezer and use a zester to grate the set amount when needed. This extends the life of the ginger and makes the ginger "fluffier." Because it expands when grating, use about 50 percent more volume than the recipe calls for.

SERVES 1   PREP TIME: **5 MINUTES**   TOTAL TIME: **5 MINUTES**

- 1½ cups water
- ½ cup unsweetened flax milk or other non-dairy milk
- 1 serving vanilla or unflavored vegetable-based protein powder
- ⅓ cup canned navy beans, with canning liquid
- 1 to 2 teaspoons grated fresh ginger
- Ground cinnamon
- ½ cup crushed ice

In a high-speed blender, combine the water, flax milk, protein powder, beans, ginger, and cinnamon. Add the ice. Blend all the ingredients until smooth.

GLUTEN-FREE OPTION: No modification needed
VEGAN OPTION: No modification needed
AIP OPTION: Use AIP-approved protein powder; omit the beans

Peppermint Nut Butter Shake

Thin Mints anyone? Here's the answer if you feel yourself due for a fix of chocolate mint anything. Cocoa itself is low in iodine, but most chocolate products have additional ingredients that are high in iodine, such as dairy items. Toasted carob works well in place of cocoa.

SERVES 1 PREP TIME: **5 MINUTES** TOTAL TIME: **5 MINUTES**

- 1½ cups water
- 2 to 3 drops peppermint extract
- 1 serving vanilla or unflavored vegetable-based protein powder
- 2 teaspoons unsweetened cocoa powder or toasted carob powder
- ⅓ cup canned navy beans, with canning liquid
- ½ teaspoon salt
- ½ tablespoon organic nut butter
- ½ cup crushed ice

In a high-speed blender, combine the water, peppermint extract, protein powder, cocoa powder, beans, salt, and nut butter. Add the ice. Blend all the ingredients until smooth.

GLUTEN-FREE OPTION: No modification needed
VEGAN OPTION: No modification needed
AIP OPTION: Use AIP-approved protein powder; use coconut yogurt instead of beans

Pumpkin Pie Delight

Pumpkin is an underutilized ingredient. Canned pumpkin is readily available and works well in this recipe. Look for versions that don't have sweeteners or salt and that are in BPA-free cans. The label says different, but when I measure, I find that each 14.5-ounce can yields almost exactly 2 cups puree.

SERVES 1   PREP TIME: **5 MINUTES**   TOTAL TIME: **5 MINUTES**

- 1½ cups unsweetened flax milk or other non-dairy milk
- 1 serving vanilla or unflavored vegetable-based protein powder
- ½ teaspoon pumpkin pie spice
- ½ cup organic pumpkin puree (not pumpkin pie filling)
- ½ organic banana, frozen, with peel
- 2 teaspoons organic honey
- ½ cup crushed ice

In a high-speed blender, combine the flax milk, protein powder, pumpkin pie spice, pumpkin puree, banana, and honey. Add the ice. Blend all the ingredients until smooth.

GLUTEN-FREE OPTION: No modification needed
VEGAN OPTION: No modification needed
AIP OPTION: Use AIP-approved protein powder

Orange Spice Shake

This is tasty and easy. Fresh orange zest is a great source of bioflavonoids, which improve thyroid hormone metabolism.

SERVES 1　　　PREP TIME: **5 MINUTES**　　　TOTAL TIME: **5 MINUTES**

- 1 cup water
- ½ cup unsweetened flax milk or other non-dairy milk
- 1 serving vanilla or unflavored vegetable-based protein powder
- ¼ teaspoon ground cinnamon
- ⅛ teaspoon ground cloves
- ⅓ cup canned navy beans, with canning liquid
- 2 teaspoons grated orange zest
- 1 medium orange, peeled and sectioned
- ½ cup crushed ice

In a high-speed blender, combine the water, flax milk, protein powder, cinnamon, cloves, beans, orange zest, and orange sections. Add the ice. Blend all the ingredients until smooth.

GLUTEN-FREE OPTION: No modification needed

VEGAN OPTION: No modification needed

AIP OPTION: Use AIP-approved protein powder; use coconut yogurt instead of beans

Apple Pie Shake

Here's one of our all-time favorite shakes. Any kind of apple works well. The raw oats are a good source of resistant starch, and unsweetened non-dairy yogurt can work well in place of the beans.

SERVES 1   **PREP TIME: 5 MINUTES**   **TOTAL TIME: 5 MINUTES**

- 1½ cups unsweetened flax milk or other non-dairy milk
- 1 serving vanilla or unflavored vegetable-based protein powder
- ⅓ cup canned navy beans, with canning liquid
- 1 Granny Smith apple, peeled and cored
- ¼ cup old-fashioned rolled oats
- 1 tablespoon chopped raw cashews
- ½ teaspoon ground Ceylon cinnamon
- ½ cup crushed ice

In a high-speed blender, combine the flax milk, protein powder, beans, apple, oats, cashews, and cinnamon. Add the ice. Blend all the ingredients until smooth.

GLUTEN-FREE OPTION: No modification needed

VEGAN OPTION: No modification needed

AIP OPTION: Use AIP-approved protein powder; use coconut yogurt instead of beans

OTHER BREAKFASTS

Easy Breakfast Oatmeal

I make this simple dish for breakfast on most days. Normally, I have some steel-cut or whole oat groats that have been batch-cooked and stored in a container. How do you know what a serving size is when you batch-cook? I usually cook 1 cup of oats at a time. When I spoon out some for a breakfast, I eyeball one-fourth of what is in the container; over four days, it averages out to be accurate. I include a little stevia when I cook the oats, so I don't need to bother adding sweetener when I assemble the breakfast.

SERVES 1   PREP TIME: **2 MINUTES**   TOTAL TIME: **5 MINUTES**

- ¼ cup cooked oatmeal
- ½ cup frozen blueberries
- 2 tablespoons raw sunflower seeds
- 1 (6-ounce) serving unflavored non-dairy yogurt
- Sweetener (optional; stevia or lo han)

Place the oatmeal and blueberries in a microwave-safe bowl. Microwave for 1 minute, or until blueberries are soft. Add the sunflower seeds, yogurt, and sweetener and stir.

GLUTEN-FREE OPTION: No modification needed
VEGAN OPTION: No modification needed
AIP OPTION: Use pumpkin puree or mashed butternut squash in place of the oatmeal

Egg White Omelet

Here is a quick and savory protein option for breakfast, or even for dinner.

SERVES 1 **PREP TIME: 5 MINUTES** **TOTAL TIME: 15 MINUTES**

- Avocado oil in a mister or nonstick cooking spray
- 3 scallions, white and green parts sliced
- 1 cup sliced fresh button mushrooms
- 1 cup liquid egg whites
- ¼ teaspoon paprika
- ⅛ to ¼ teaspoon ground turmeric
- ½ teaspoon toasted sesame oil

1. Place a small skillet on medium heat and mist with the avocado oil.
2. Sauté the scallion whites and the mushrooms for 2 to 3 minutes or until soft. Transfer to a plate.
3. Increase the heat under the skillet to medium high. Add the egg whites, stir in the paprika, then slowly stir in the turmeric until the eggs are light yellow.
4. Cook the egg whites 1 to 2 minutes, until just firm. Drizzle on the sesame oil and transfer to the plate with the scallions and mushrooms. Sprinkle on the scallion greens and serve.

GLUTEN-FREE OPTION: No modification needed
VEGAN OPTION: Use soft tofu or other plant-based egg product
AIP OPTION: No option available

Three-Ingredient Pancakes

When is it time to make these pancakes? Any time you have some bananas sitting around, getting overripe! If desired, top the pancakes with berries and serve with non-dairy yogurt or a protein shake to get more protein. Rather than commercial cooking spray, I like to use avocado oil (or other heat-stable oil) in a hand misting bottle.

SERVES 2　　　　PREP TIME: **2 MINUTES**　　　　TOTAL TIME: **10 MINUTES**

- 2 ripe bananas, peeled
- 1 cup old-fashioned rolled oats
- ½ cup liquid egg whites
- Avocado oil in a mister or nonstick cooking spray

1. In a medium bowl, use a fork to mash the bananas. Add the oats and egg whites to the bowl and mix well.
2. Coat a griddle or large skillet with a misting of the avocado oil. Heat over medium-high heat until hot enough to sizzle a drop of water.
3. Reduce the heat to medium, then scoop the batter, using a ¼ cup measure, onto the griddle, leaving ½ inch space between the pancakes.
4. Cook for 2 minutes, then flip and cook for another minute, until the pancakes are lightly browned. Serve at once.

SERVING SUGGESTION: Add additional protein for complete protein serving
GLUTEN-FREE OPTION: No modification needed
VEGAN OPTION: Omit the egg whites and replace with 1 serving pea protein powder
AIP OPTION: Omit the egg whites and replace the oats with shredded coconut

Sweet Potato Hash

This is my go-to recipe for a breakfast hash. You can use an old-fashioned box shredder or a food processor to shred the veggies here. There are few limits to what you can include for the veggies and protein in this dish!

SERVES 4   PREP TIME: 15 MINUTES   TOTAL TIME: 25 MINUTES

- Avocado oil in a mister or nonstick cooking spray
- 2 sweet potatoes, peeled and shredded
- 1 medium zucchini, shredded
- 1 small white onion, shredded
- 1 cup liquid egg whites
- Salt and freshly ground black pepper

1. Mist a large skillet with the avocado oil and place over medium-high heat. Spread the sweet potatoes in the skillet, then reduce the heat to medium, cover the skillet, and cook for 3 minutes.
2. Add the zucchini and onion, stir, cover again, and cook for 3 more minutes.
3. Raise the heat to high, then add the egg whites, stirring and cooking until set, about 1 minute. Season to taste with salt and pepper, then serve.

SERVING SUGGESTION: Add a side of chicken or use extra egg whites for complete protein

GLUTEN-FREE OPTION: No modification needed

VEGAN OPTION: Replace the egg whites with ½ block firm tofu, crumbled

AIP OPTION: Replace the egg whites with diced cooked meat of choice

Buckwheat Berry Porridge

If you love oats, you are in for a real treat with buckwheat. For this recipe, you'll want raw buckwheat groats. If you don't mind taking an extra minute, they come out even better with a light toasting before cooking. Just heat them over medium heat in a dry skillet until they just barely darken and become fragrant. This is a great recipe to batch-cook and refrigerate for later.

SERVES 4   **PREP TIME: 3 MINUTES**   **TOTAL TIME: 20 MINUTES**

- 1 cup buckwheat groats
- 1 cinnamon stick
- 1½ cups unflavored non-dairy milk (I use unsweetened flax milk)
- 1 cup fresh blackberries
- ¼ cup raw, unsalted pumpkin seeds

1. Place the buckwheat, cinnamon stick, non-dairy milk, 1½ cups water, the blackberries, and the pumpkin seeds in a medium saucepan and bring to a low simmer over medium heat.
2. Lightly cover and simmer for 15 minutes. The buckwheat should have the texture of a hearty porridge. Let rest for 5 minutes, then remove the cinnamon stick and serve.

SERVING SUGGESTION: Serve with a side of protein to make a complete breakfast
GLUTEN-FREE OPTION: No modification needed
VEGAN OPTION: No modification needed
AIP OPTION: No option available

Vanilla Millet Hot Cereal

Millet makes one of the quickest-cooking hot cereals and it has a texture akin to mashed potatoes. It is an excellent source of copper and magnesium. This is a great recipe to batch-cook.

SERVES 4 **PREP TIME: 5 MINUTES** **TOTAL TIME: 25 MINUTES**

- 1 cup whole millet
- 1 teaspoon natural vanilla extract or other flavoring
- 1 medium pear, cored and diced
- ¼ cup almonds, chopped
- Sweetener of choice (stevia or lo han)

1. Place the millet, vanilla, pear, almonds, sweetener, and 2½ cups water in a medium saucepan.
2. Bring to a boil over high heat, then reduce the heat and simmer for 20 minutes, lightly covered, until the mixture firms up into a hearty porridge. Let sit for 5 minutes, then serve.

SERVING SUGGESTION: Serve with non-dairy milk; for a complete breakfast, serve with a side of protein

GLUTEN-FREE OPTION: No modification needed

VEGAN OPTION: No modification needed

AIP OPTION: No option available

Huevos Rancheros

Remember that egg whites are a safe food choice and you can do so much with them! Watch your energy levels throughout the day after having this meal for breakfast—you may find they are steadier than normal, and your blood sugar will be more stable after the day's other meals, as well. If you don't have cooked potatoes on hand, you can quickly cook one in the microwave; just peel it, jab a fork into it several times, and heat on full power for 3 to 5 minutes. You'll have as much resistant starch present as if you had boiled the potato.

SERVES 2   PREP TIME: 10 MINUTES   TOTAL TIME: 20 MINUTES

- Avocado oil in a mister or nonstick cooking spray
- ¼ cup diced onion
- 2 cups liquid egg whites (or whites from 12 large eggs)
- 1 boiled medium potato, peeled and cut into bite-size pieces
- 1 Roma (plum) tomato, cored and diced
- 1 cup canned pinto beans
- 2 cups fresh spinach
- ½ avocado, diced
- ¼ cup fresh cilantro, minced
- Salt and freshly ground black pepper
- Hot sauce of choice (optional)

1. Mist a large skillet with the avocado oil and heat over high heat until a drop of water sizzles.
2. Add the onion and sauté for 1 to 2 minutes, until translucent. Add the egg whites and sauté an additional minute, or until the whites have mostly firmed up.
3. Add the potato, tomato, beans, and spinach. Sauté for 3 to 4 minutes, until the spinach is wilted.
4. Transfer to plates and garnish with the avocado and cilantro, then season with salt and pepper, and serve with hot sauce, if desired.

GLUTEN-FREE OPTION: No modification needed
VEGAN OPTION: Substitute ½ block of firm tofu for the egg whites
AIP OPTION: No option available

Pecan-Banana Teff Cereal

Teff is a staple food in Ethiopia, but it is rarely used in the States. Besides being tasty (kind of like cocoa cream of wheat), it is rich in iron and resistant starch. Most larger health food supermarkets have it. If you can't find it, steel-cut oats work great in this recipe, also. Refrigerate any leftovers and serve the next day.

SERVES 4   **PREP TIME: 5 MINUTES**   **TOTAL TIME: 25 MINUTES**

- 1 cup whole-grain teff
- 1 cup unsweetened flax milk
- ¼ cup crushed pecans
- 1 banana, peeled and diced
- ½ teaspoon ground cinnamon

Combine the teff, 2 cups water, the flax milk, pecans, banana, and cinnamon in a large saucepan. Bring to a low simmer over medium heat. Simmer for 25 minutes, stirring occasionally. Serve.

SERVING SUGGESTION: Serve with a side of protein to make a complete breakfast
GLUTEN-FREE OPTION: No modification needed
VEGAN OPTION: No modification needed
AIP OPTION: No option available

Whole Oat Porridge

This is a nice way to use whole oats, also called oat groats. Each time a grain is broken, as in processing, some flavors are lost and some of the oils oxidize. Using whole grains may be important for the preservation of beneficial phytonutrients. In terms of fiber, protein, vitamins, and minerals, whole oats and processed oats are pretty much identical in all other forms. Think of it as a continuum from the least oxidized to the most: whole, steel-cut, old-fashioned rolled, regular rolled, quick-cooking, and instant oats. Mind you, if I am traveling or short on staples, I'll take instant oats over donuts for breakfast any day. When I have time, though, whole oats are my favorite.

SERVES 8 PREP TIME: 2 MINUTES TOTAL TIME: 4 TO 6 HOURS IN A SLOW COOKER

- 8 cups purified water
- 2 cups whole oats or steel-cut oats
- 2 to 3 cinnamon sticks
- Optional flavorings:
  1 teaspoon ground cloves
  1 tablespoon ground cardamom

Place the water, oats, and cinnamon sticks in a slow cooker; add the desired flavorings. Close the cooker and cook on the low setting for 4 to 6 hours. Open the cooker and remove the cinnamon sticks. Serve.

SERVING SUGGESTION: Mix in protein powder or serve with egg whites for a complete meal; top with fresh fruit—apples and pears work well

GLUTEN-FREE OPTION: No modification needed

VEGAN OPTION: No modification needed

AIP OPTION: In a high-speed blender, combine 1½ cups tigernuts, 1 cup coconut flakes, and ½ cup konjac root powder; blend until the pieces are as small as instant oats, then use in place of the oats and reduce the water to 6 cups

Brazil Nut Quickbread

This can be part of your breakfast, or a good-carb side dish for dinner. The citrus flavors work nicely with the Brazil nuts.

SERVES 6 **PREP TIME: 20 MINUTES** **TOTAL TIME: 60 MINUTES**

- Avocado oil in a mister or nonstick cooking spray
- ⅓ cup white whole wheat flour
- 2 teaspoons toasted carob powder or unsweetened cocoa powder
- ½ teaspoon ground cinnamon
- ½ teaspoon baking powder
- ½ teaspoon salt
- ¾ cup liquid egg whites or egg substitute
- 2 tablespoons unflavored non-dairy milk
- 1 tablespoon grated orange zest
- ¾ cup chopped Brazil nuts
- 1 cup chopped pitted Medjool dates

1. Preheat the oven to 325°F. Mist a 4 by 8-inch baking pan with the avocado oil.
2. Combine the flour, carob powder, cinnamon, baking powder, and salt in a large bowl.
3. Stir in the egg whites, non-dairy milk, zest, nuts, and dates. Mix well, until the batter is smooth.
4. Pour the batter into the baking pan and bake for 40 minutes, until the top is lightly browned and the center pushes back. Cool on a rack, then slice and serve.

SERVING SUGGESTION: Add a side of protein for a complete meal
GLUTEN-FREE OPTION: Use gluten-free baking mix instead of the whole wheat flour
VEGAN OPTION: Use egg substitute
AIP OPTION: No option available

Overnight Apple Pie Oats

Do you have a busy morning coming up? It takes all of five minutes to put this together. You can serve all of it at once or refrigerate unused portions for up to four days.

SERVES 8   PREP TIME: **10 MINUTES**   TOTAL TIME: **24 HOURS**

- 2 cups old-fashioned rolled oats
- 2 small to medium apples (Gala or Pink Lady), cored and chopped
- 1 teaspoon ground Ceylon cinnamon
- 2 cups unsweetened flax milk or other non-dairy milk
- 4 teaspoons chia seeds

Combine the oats, apples, cinnamon, flax milk, and chia seeds in a large bowl. Refrigerate overnight. Serve.

SERVING SUGGESTION: Add a side of protein for a complete meal

GLUTEN-FREE OPTION: No modification needed

VEGAN OPTION: No modification needed

AIP OPTION: Use cooked and cubed butternut squash instead of oats; omit dairy substitute

Buckwheat Banana Bread

Here is another good use for overripe bananas. It also helps you work in your buckwheat and Brazil nuts for the day. The bread keeps for a few days, but don't expect it to last if you have a family around. If you don't have buckwheat flour, you can blend 1⅔ cups of dry buckwheat groats in a blender to make the flour.

SERVES 10 **PREP TIME: 15 MINUTES** **TOTAL TIME: 75 MINUTES**

- 1½ cups buckwheat flour
- 1 teaspoon baking soda
- ¼ teaspoon salt
- 2 teaspoons ground Ceylon cinnamon
- 3 very ripe bananas, peeled
- ½ cup liquid egg whites
- ⅓ cup honey or safe sweetener of your choice
- ½ cup unsweetened flax milk
- ½ cup chopped Brazil nuts
- 2 teaspoons pure vanilla extract

1. Preheat the oven to 350° F. Line a 9 by 5-inch loaf pan with parchment paper.
2. In a small bowl, mix the flour, baking soda, salt, and cinnamon. Whisk until evenly blended.
3. In a large bowl, mash the bananas with the egg whites, using a fork. Add the sweetener, flax milk, Brazil nuts, and vanilla. Mix well.
4. Pour the flour mixture into the banana mixture and mix until all the flour is incorporated. The batter will be thin and chunky.
5. Pour the batter into the loaf pan and bake for 60 to 70 minutes, or until a toothpick stuck in the center of the loaf comes out dry. Let cool on a rack for 30 minutes, then remove from the pan, slice, and serve.

SERVING SUGGESTION: Can be served with a protein for a quick breakfast or as a good carb for lunch and dinner

GLUTEN-FREE OPTION: No modification needed

VEGAN OPTION: Use 2 tablespoons Egg Replacer powder instead of the eggs; combine with ¾ cup water, mix well, and add the remaining ingredients

AIP OPTION: Substitute cassava flour for the buckwheat flour

SALADS, BOWLS, AND WRAPS

Freekeh Tabbouleh

Besides being a fun word to say (free-Kah), freekeh is among the lowest-glycemic good carbs. It is slower to digest because it is harvested before it is completely ripe. This also leaves it higher in pigmented phytonutrients like lutein and zeaxanthin.

SERVES 4   **PREP TIME: 15 MINUTES**   **TOTAL TIME: 20 MINUTES**

- ½ teaspoon salt
- 1 cup cracked freekeh, rinsed and drained
- 1 lemon, zested and juiced
- 2 teaspoons extra-virgin olive oil
- 1 cup fresh parsley, large stems removed and leaves finely chopped
- 1 medium red onion, finely diced
- 3 ripe Roma (plum) tomatoes, seeded and chopped
- 1 medium cucumber, peeled and seeded
- 1 cup green grapes, halved
- 4 Medjool dates, pitted and chopped
- ¼ cup sunflower seeds

1. Place 1½ cups water in a small saucepan set over high heat and bring to a boil. Add the salt and freekeh, reduce the heat to low, and simmer until tender, about 15 minutes.
2. Drain the freekeh, then spread out on a baking sheet and place in the refrigerator to quickly cool.
3. Combine the chilled freekeh with the lemon zest and juice, olive oil, parsley, red onion, tomatoes, cucumber, grapes, dates, and sunflower seeds. Serve.

SERVING SUGGESTION: Serve with leftover protein for a complete meal
GLUTEN-FREE OPTION: Replace the freekeh with quinoa
VEGAN OPTION: No modification needed
AIP OPTION: Replace the freekeh with riced zucchini

Mediterranean Fennel Salad

Fennel shares with licorice and anise a volatile oil called anethole. The fennel bulb is tough and fibrous. It is a member of the Apiaceae family, along with carrots, parsley, celery, and parsnips. This group of plants is uniquely beneficial to liver function. To use fennel raw in a salad, you shave it into very thin slices.

SERVES 4 **PREP TIME: 20 MINUTES** **TOTAL TIME: 20 MINUTES**

FOR THE SALAD

- 1 head romaine lettuce, torn into bite-size pieces
- 1 small fennel bulb, outer leaves discarded, bulb cut into thin slices
- ½ small red onion, sliced
- 1 (14-ounce) BPA-free, no salt added can artichoke hearts in water, drained and cut into quarters
- 1 (14.5-ounce) BPA-free, no salt added can chickpeas, drained and with liquid reserved
- 2 ripe Roma (plum) tomatoes, diced
- 1 jar (at least 4 ounces) pitted Kalamata olives. Take ⅓ cup olives and dice
- 1 medium cucumber, peeled, seeded, and sliced

FOR THE DRESSING

- 2 tablespoons extra-virgin olive oil
- 1 teaspoon nutritional yeast (with no synthetic folic acid)
- 3 tablespoons red wine vinegar
- 2 teaspoons stone-ground mustard
- 1 teaspoon herbes de Provence
- Salt and freshly ground black pepper

1. Place all the salad ingredients in a large bowl.
2. In a small bowl, combine the dressing ingredients with ½ cup of liquid from the chickpeas. Mix well.
3. Pour the dressing over the salad and toss. Serve immediately.

SERVING SUGGESTION: Serve with a side of protein for a complete meal
GLUTEN-FREE OPTION: No modification needed
VEGAN OPTION: No modification needed
AIP OPTION: Omit tomatoes, vinegar, yeast, and chickpeas

Classic Niçoise Salad

Kirin is famous for her Niçoise salad. It is one of the few salad meals that fills me up. By peeling the potatoes, and by using only the egg whites, it's easy to make this meal low in iodine.

SERVES 4 **PREP TIME: 25 MINUTES** **TOTAL TIME: 30 MINUTES**

FOR THE SALAD

- 1 (12.5-ounce) can chicken breast, drained
- 9 hard-boiled eggs, peeled and quartered, yolks discarded
- 1 pound Yukon Gold potatoes (2 to 3 medium), quartered and cooked until fork-tender (5 to 8 minutes)
- 2 heads butter lettuce, torn into small pieces
- 1 pint ripe cherry tomatoes, halved
- 1 medium red onion, thinly sliced
- 8 ounces green beans, cut into 2-inch pieces, blanched for 4 minutes
- ¼ cup pitted kalamata olives
- 2 tablespoons rinsed capers
- 2 teaspoons nutritional yeast (folic-acid-free)

FOR THE DRESSING

- ⅓ cup lemon juice or red wine vinegar
- ¾ cup extra-virgin olive oil
- 3 tablespoons finely chopped shallots
- 2 tablespoons finely chopped fresh basil
- 1 tablespoon finely chopped fresh thyme
- 2 teaspoons finely chopped fresh oregano or tarragon
- 1 teaspoon Dijon mustard
- Salt and freshly ground black pepper

Combine the salad ingredients in a large bowl. Combine the dressing ingredients in a jar, shake well, then drizzle over the salad and toss well.

SERVING SUGGESTION: Salad ingredients can be made several hours in advance, covered, and refrigerated until ready to serve

GLUTEN-FREE OPTION: No modification needed

VEGAN OPTION: Omit the tuna

AIP OPTION: Omit the potatoes and tomatoes

Healthy Caesar Salad

I love Caesar salads, but it seems like restaurants try their best to turn them into bombs of empty calories. If you want a lighter lunch that can be assembled in just a few moments, this fits the bill. This recipe does call for two moderate-iodine foods (anchovies and parmesan), but the amounts used are less than one-fourth a typical serving. Cabbage is not a traditional ingredient, but it lends a crunchy texture to the salad.

SERVES 4 **PREP TIME: 10 MINUTES** **TOTAL TIME: 10 MINUTES**

- 3 cups (½-inch) cubes of whole-grain sourdough bread (optional; see page 232)
- Avocado oil in a mister (optional)
- 2 to 3 garlic cloves, minced
- Salt and freshly ground black pepper
- 2 heads romaine lettuce, torn into bite-size pieces
- 2 cups shredded green cabbage
- 1 tablespoon minced fresh parsley
- 2 teaspoons sherry vinegar
- 1 teaspoon Dijon mustard
- 1 teaspoon minced fresh thyme leaves, or ½ teaspoon mixed dried herbs
- 1 tablespoon extra-virgin olive oil
- 2 anchovy fillets, rinsed, dried, and mashed
- 1 tablespoon grated parmesan cheese

1. If making the croutons, preheat the oven to 350°F. Place the bread cubes in a small bowl, mist with the avocado oil or drizzle on about 1 teaspoon, then stir in one-third of the garlic and add salt and pepper. Spread the croutons on a baking sheet and bake for 10 minutes, stirring halfway through to crisp all sides. Let cool briefly.

2. Arrange the lettuce and cabbage in 4 serving bowls.

3. Whisk together the remaining garlic, the parsley, vinegar, mustard, thyme, olive oil, and anchovies into a thick dressing.

4. Pour the dressing over the lettuce, garnish each bowl with some croutons if using, and sprinkle with the parmesan.

SERVING SUGGESTION: Serve with a light protein dish and more sourdough bread or with a side of warmed cannellini beans

GLUTEN-FREE OPTION: No modification needed

VEGAN OPTION: Replace the anchovies with 2 teaspoons tamari; replace the cheese with 2 teaspoons nutritional yeast

AIP OPTION: Omit the croutons; replace the cheese with 2 teaspoons nutritional yeast

Chai Potato Bowl

Here is a dish to make in advance so you have a ready-to-go lunch the next day. Chai seasoning is a mixture of spices I like to have on hand for general use; it includes cinnamon, cardamom, cloves, ginger, and black pepper. I modified the classic chai combo to be lighter on the sweetest seasonings, the cinnamon and cardamom. I use purple potatoes here; red or gold potatoes would also work.

SERVES 2　　　PREP TIME: **10 MINUTES**　　　TOTAL TIME: **65 MINUTES**

- 1 teaspoon coarse salt
- 1 teaspoon freshly ground black pepper
- 1 teaspoon ground ginger
- ½ teaspoon ground Ceylon cinnamon
- ½ teaspoon ground cardamom
- ⅛ teaspoon ground cloves
- 2 purple potatoes, peeled and cubed
- 2 (6-ounce) skinless boneless chicken breasts, diced
- Avocado oil in a mister or nonstick cooking spray
- 4 cups fresh spinach

1. Preheat the oven to 400°F. Line a baking sheet with parchment paper or a silicone mat.

2. In a small bowl, combine the salt, pepper, ginger, cinnamon, cardamom, and cloves.

3. In a medium bowl, combine the potatoes with half the seasoning blend and stir to lightly coat. Spread the potatoes on the baking sheet and bake until fork-tender, about 45 minutes.

4. Place the chicken in a medium bowl and sprinkle with the remaining seasoning mix; stir to coat well.

5. Mist a large skillet with some avocado oil. Heat over medium heat, then add the chicken and sauté until cooked through and lightly browned, 3 to 5 minutes, turning often so the seasonings do not burn.

6. Add the spinach to the skillet and stir until the leaves have wilted, about 3 minutes.

7. Transfer the chicken and spinach to serving bowls and add some of the roasted potatoes to each. Serve.

GLUTEN-FREE OPTION: No modification needed

VEGAN OPTION: Replace the chicken with extra-firm tofu

AIP OPTION: Replace the potatoes with roasted beets, baking instead for 25 minutes

Cilantro Shrimp Bowl

Shrimp is a moderate-iodine food, but the iodine levels are acceptably low when the shrimp is boiled. That's because iodine is water-soluble, so much of it is lost in contact with water. Also, shrimp purchased without its shells is lower in iodine.

SERVES 4 **PREP TIME: 15 MINUTES** **TOTAL TIME: 30 MINUTES**

- 2 tablespoons salt
- 1 pound peeled and deveined medium shrimp, cut into thirds
- 1 (14.5-ounce) BPA-free can, no salt added black beans, drained and with liquid reserved
- 1 bunch scallions, white and green parts cut into ¼-inch pieces
- 1 medium avocado, peeled, seeded, and diced
- 1 ripe beefsteak tomato, cored and diced
- 1 loose head red-leaf lettuce, torn into small pieces
- 1 bunch fresh cilantro, chopped
- 2 garlic cloves
- 1 teaspoon ground cumin
- Juice of 2 limes

1. Place about 2 quarts of water in a medium saucepan and bring to a boil. Add the salt and shrimp, reduce the heat, and simmer for 5 minutes. Drain thoroughly.

2. In a large salad bowl, combine the shrimp, beans, scallions, avocado, and tomato. Add the lettuce and toss.

3. In a small blender or food processor, combine the cilantro, garlic, cumin, lime juice, and ½ cup liquid from the beans. Blend the dressing until smooth.

4. Pour the dressing over the salad ingredients and stir. Serve immediately.

GLUTEN-FREE OPTION: No modification needed
VEGAN OPTION: Omit the shrimp or replace with cubed dried seasoned tofu
AIP OPTION: Omit the beans and tomatoes or replace with 1 cup cubed cooked squash

Ceviche Salad

Here is another great way to perfectly "cook" seafood. The acid from the lemon juice changes the protein in a way similar to heat, so the seafood is technically not raw anymore. But watch: it can become too tough if it sits in the acid for longer than recommended.

SERVES 4 PREP TIME: **30 MINUTES** TOTAL TIME: **45 MINUTES**

FOR THE SALAD

- 1 loose head red-leaf lettuce, finely chopped
- 1 avocado, peeled, seeded, and diced
- 2 ripe beefsteak tomatoes, cored and diced
- 2 tablespoons pumpkin seeds
- 1 (14.5-ounce) BPA-free, no salt added can cannellini beans, drained
- 1 teaspoon dried tarragon, or 1 tablespoon chopped fresh

FOR THE CEVICHE

- 1 pound lower-iodine seafood of choice (catfish, flounder, halibut or scallops), cut into small dice
- ¾ cup fresh lime juice
- ¼ cup fresh lemon juice
- 1 teaspoon salt
- ⅓ cup chopped fresh cilantro
- ½ medium red onion, diced
- 2 tablespoons extra-virgin olive oil
- Freshly ground black pepper

1. Mix the salad ingredients in a serving bowl.
2. Thoroughly mix the ceviche ingredients in a medium bowl. Refrigerate for 10 minutes, then let sit at room temperature for 10 minutes.
3. Pour off roughly half the liquid from the ceviche, then add the ceviche and remaining liquid to the salad. Toss and serve.

SERVING SUGGESTION: Serve with a side of carbs for a complete meal

GLUTEN-FREE OPTION: No modification needed

VEGAN OPTION: Use extra-firm tofu instead of the seafood; place the diced tofu between layers of paper toweling, weighted down with a heavy pan for 10 minutes before soaking in the ceviche liquid

AIP OPTION: Omit the tomatoes and replace the beans with cauliflower florets; serve with a side of carbs

Shiitake Soba Bowl

Here is another great way to get the benefits of buckwheat, which is among the densest food sources of polyphenols and bioflavonoids. These soba noodles are also fast to cook, usually 2 to 3 minutes. Dried shiitakes are easy to find online or in specialty grocery stores; I love them because of their shelf life and their price point, but you can use fresh as well. If you use dried, just soak them in room-temperature water for 20 minutes before starting the recipe.

SERVES 4 **PREP TIME: 30 MINUTES** **TOTAL TIME: 30 MINUTES**

- 1 navel orange, peeled and sectioned
- 3 teaspoons miso paste
- 2 garlic cloves, crushed
- 2 tablespoons red wine vinegar
- 1 tablespoon toasted sesame oil
- 2 teaspoons avocado oil
- 1 pound fresh or soaked dried shiitake mushrooms, sliced
- 3 baby bok choy, sliced, white stems separated from leaves
- 2 cups sugar snap peas, trimmed
- 1 red bell pepper, cored, seeded, and sliced into matchstick pieces
- 4 young bulbing onions, sliced lengthwise into 4 pieces, then cut into 1-inch lengths
- 1 (8-ounce) package soba noodles, cooked
- 1 pound cooked chicken or extra-firm tofu, diced

1. In a blender, combine the orange, miso, garlic, vinegar, and sesame oil. Pour through a strainer into a small bowl.
2. Heat the avocado oil in a wok or large skillet over medium-high heat. Add the mushrooms and bok choy stems, then stir-fry over high heat for 2 minutes.
3. Add the peas, bell pepper, and onions. Stir-fry an additional 2 minutes.
4. Add the noodles, chicken, and strained sauce. Stir and cook for an additional minute. Serve.

GLUTEN-FREE OPTION: No modification needed
VEGAN OPTION: Use tofu instead of chicken
AIP OPTION: Use zucchini noodles instead of the soba

Roman Wraps

Lunch on the go can be much easier than people think. Wraps are portable and can let you repurpose leftovers in a new way. But what do you put your traveling wrap inside of? Lettuce works great, but it can be messy. Try using parchment paper around the lettuce and roll it back as you eat the wrap. If you open it without tearing, it may even be able to be reused. I've found that butter lettuce has the perfect combination of flavor, pliability, and structural stability to work as a wrap container. Romaine is a decent second option. Be sure to wash and thoroughly dry your lettuce leaves first. Too much moisture can make them adhere to the parchment paper. You'll need four pieces of parchment, each measuring roughly 10 inches square.

SERVES 2 (MAKES 4 WRAPS) PREP TIME: **5 MINUTES**   TOTAL TIME: **5 MINUTES**

- ½ head butter lettuce, leaves removed and stacked (16 leaves)
- 1 (8- to 10-ounce) skinless boneless chicken breast, cooked and sliced
- 1 handful of arugula, trimmed
- 2 ripe Roma (plum) tomatoes, cored and thinly sliced
- ¼ medium red onion, thinly sliced
- ½ cup no salt added canned cannellini beans
- 1 teaspoon Italian seasoning blend
- Balsamic vinegar or glaze
- Extra-virgin olive oil

1. For each wrap, place 4 large lettuce leaves overlapping on a sheet of parchment paper that measures roughly 10 inches square.
2. Add one-fourth of the chicken, arugula, tomatoes, red onion, balsamic, olive oil, beans and salt and pepper to taste.
3. Fold over one end of the paper, then roll up, encasing the contents. Repeat with the remaining leaves and ingredients to make 3 more wraps.

SERVING SUGGESTION: This can be a stand-alone meal, or you can include additional snacking vegetables

GLUTEN-FREE OPTION: No modification needed

VEGAN OPTION: Omit the chicken or replace with sliced seasoned dried tofu

AIP OPTION: Omit the cannellini beans

Masala Lentil Wraps

This wrap lends itself to lots of adaptation. I use fresh lentils more often than canned because they cook so quickly. All you need to do is rinse them, place in a saucepan, cover with 2 to 3 inches of water, and simmer for about 20 minutes. I usually cook a pound at a time and keep some in the refrigerator for later use. Lentils are higher in protein than other legumes, but not high enough for your full serving of protein, so I add one serving of protein to have with this. You'll need four pieces of parchment paper, each measuring roughly 10 inches square.

SERVES 4 (MAKES 4 WRAPS)   **PREP TIME: 10 MINUTES**   **TOTAL TIME: 20 MINUTES**

- Avocado oil in a mister or nonstick cooking spray
- 1 medium yellow or sweet onion, diced
- 3 garlic cloves, crushed
- 2 teaspoons grated fresh ginger
- 1 tablespoon garam masala
- 1 teaspoon ground cumin
- 3 cups cauliflower florets, broken into small pieces (from 1 small head)
- 2 tablespoons unsalted tomato paste
- 1 (14-ounce) BPA-free can, no salt added lentils, rinsed and drained
- 1 (14-ounce) BPA-free can unsalted diced tomatoes, drained
- 1 head butter lettuce, leaves removed and stacked (16 leaves)
- ¼ cup fresh cilantro, chopped
- Salt and freshly ground black pepper

1. Mist a large skillet with the avocado oil and heat over medium-high heat until hot enough that a drop of water sizzles.

2. Add the onion and sauté until translucent, 2 to 3 minutes. Add the garlic, ginger, garam masala, and cumin and sauté an additional 30 seconds.

3. Add the cauliflower, tomato paste, lentils, and tomatoes to the skillet. Stir, cooking, until the cauliflower is softened, about 5 minutes.

4. Place 4 large lettuce leaves overlapping on a sheet of parchment paper that measures roughly 10 inches square.

5. Add one-fourth of the mixture, then sprinkle on the cilantro and season with salt and pepper.

6. Fold over one end of the parchment paper, then roll up, encasing the contents. Repeat with the remaining ingredients to make 3 more wraps.

SERVING SUGGESTION: Add 1 serving of protein for a complete meal; you can also include snacking vegetables

GLUTEN-FREE OPTION: No modification needed

VEGAN OPTION: No modification needed

AIP OPTION: No option available

Sesame Ginger Lettuce Wraps

Asian seasonings rely heavily on fish sauce, so takeout dishes often have unsafe levels of iodine. The core Asian flavors come from tamari, toasted sesame oil, rice vinegar, garlic, and ginger, so these can be combined with many ingredients for delicious homemade Asian dishes that are low in iodine. You'll need four pieces of parchment paper, each measuring roughly 10 inches square.

SERVES 4 (MAKES 4 WRAPS)   **PREP TIME: 10 MINUTES**   **TOTAL TIME: 20 MINUTES**

- Avocado oil in a mister or nonstick cooking spray
- ½ medium yellow or sweet onion, diced
- 1 pound lean ground beef
- 8 ounces snow peas
- 1 (12-ounce) package udon noodles, cooked according to package directions
- 2 tablespoons tamari
- 2 garlic cloves, crushed
- 2 teaspoons grated fresh ginger
- 1 teaspoon toasted sesame oil
- 2 tablespoons rice vinegar
- 1 head butter lettuce, leaves removed and stacked (16 leaves)

1. Mist a large skillet with some avocado oil and heat over medium-high heat until hot enough that a drop of water will sizzle.

2. Add the onion and sauté until translucent, roughly 2 minutes. Add the ground beef and sauté until it browns, about 4 minutes.

3. Add the snow peas and sauté an additional 2 minutes. Add the noodles, tamari, garlic, ginger, sesame oil, and vinegar and stir to blend well.

4. Place 4 large lettuce leaves overlapping on a sheet of parchment paper that measures roughly 10 inches square. Add one-fourth of the mixture to the wrap.

5. Fold over one end of the parchment paper, then roll up, encasing the contents. Repeat with the remaining ingredients to make 3 additional wraps.

SERVING SUGGESTION: This can be a stand-alone meal, or you can include additional snacking vegetables

GLUTEN-FREE OPTION: No modification needed

VEGAN OPTION: Omit the ground meat; can replace with crumbled tempeh

AIP OPTION: Omit the tamari

Southwest Scramble Wraps

Even if you're not vegan, tofu is a good source of protein, phytonutrients, calcium, and magnesium. For anything other than smoothies, I prefer extra-firm tofu. Most brands are refrigerated and in the dairy section; be sure to check the ingredients, because a few of them can have seaweed-based texturizers like carrageenan, alginates, or agar—all of which you want to avoid. You'll need four pieces of parchment paper, each measuring roughly 10 inches square.

SERVES 2 (MAKES 4 WRAPS) PREP TIME: **10 MINUTES**   TOTAL TIME: **20 MINUTES**

- Avocado oil in a mister or nonstick cooking spray
- ½ yellow or sweet onion, sliced
- 1 block extra-firm tofu, cut into bite-size cubes
- 1 or 2 garlic cloves, minced
- 1 teaspoon ground cumin
- 2 teaspoons smoked paprika
- ½ teaspoon cayenne pepper
- ½ teaspoon dried oregano
- Juice of ½ lime
- ½ (14.5-ounce) BPA-free, no salt added can black beans, drained
- 1 ripe tomato, cored and diced
- ½ head butter lettuce, leaves removed and stacked (16 leaves)

1. Mist a large skillet with the avocado oil and heat over medium-high heat until hot enough that a drop of water sizzles.
2. Add the onion and sauté until translucent, about 2 minutes. Add the tofu and sauté until browned, about 3 minutes.
3. Add the garlic, cumin, paprika, cayenne, and oregano and sauté an additional 30 seconds. Stir in the lime juice, beans, and tomato and stir well.
4. Place 4 large lettuce leaves overlapping on a sheet of parchment paper that is roughly 10 inches square.
5. Add one-fourth of the mixture to the wrap. Fold over one end of the parchment paper, then roll up. Continue to make the remaining 3 wraps.

GLUTEN-FREE OPTION: No modification needed
VEGAN OPTION: No modification needed
AIP OPTION: Replace the tofu with cooked lean beef stew or ground pork

SOUPS AND STEWS

Sweet Corn and Sorghum Soup

Here is an easy one-pot meal that is a great use for sweet corn. For those seeking to avoid GMO products, look for organic sweet corn or purchase from farmers' markets, and confirm with the farmer. This dish is also a good way to get introduced to sorghum, a gluten-free grain popular in the U.S. South. Historically, much of it was used for syrup production, but the grain is a nice chewy addition to many dishes.

SERVES 4   **PREP TIME: 15 MINUTES**   **TOTAL TIME: 1 HOUR, 45 MINUTES**

- 4 (6-ounce) skinless boneless chicken breasts
- 1 medium onion, diced
- ¾ cup sorghum grain
- 1 cup corn kernels (from about 2 ears)
- 1 (3-inch) piece fresh ginger, peeled and minced
- 3 tablespoons tamari
- 2 teaspoons chopped fresh chives, or 1 teaspoon dried
- ½ cup chopped fresh cilantro

1. Place the chicken in a large saucepan along with the onion and 2 cups water.
2. Bring to a boil over high heat, then reduce the heat to medium low and simmer for 20 minutes.
3. Add the sorghum and simmer for another 35 to 40 minutes, or until the grains are tender.
4. Add the corn, ginger, tamari, and chives. Simmer an additional 5 minutes, then sprinkle with the cilantro and serve.

GLUTEN-FREE OPTION: No modification needed
VEGAN OPTION: Substitute tofu, seitan, or meat substitute for the chicken
AIP OPTION: Omit the sorghum; replace the corn with diced mushrooms

Dr. Khoshaba's Lentil Soup

Dr. Linda Khoshaba, the medical director at our clinic, Integrative Health, invited us to dinner at her home one evening, and she served this. It's a family recipe that has been passed down through generations, and once you taste it, you'll see why. The flavor is incredible! It's filling, delicious, and even children love it. Lentils are higher in protein than other legumes, but not high enough for a complete meal serving of protein, so accompany with ½ to 1 serving of protein.

SERVES 4 TO 6   PREP TIME: **5 TO 10 MINUTES**   TOTAL TIME: **35 MINUTES**

- 1 tablespoon extra-virgin olive oil
- 1 large onion, finely chopped
- 3 tablespoons unsalted chicken or vegetable broth
- 2 cups orange lentils
- 2 teaspoons ground turmeric
- 2 teaspoons curry powder
- ½ teaspoon freshly ground black pepper
- ½ cup white rice (optional; add 1 cup water if using)

1. Place the olive oil in a large saucepan and heat over medium-low heat. Add the onion and sauté about 5 minutes, until almost caramelized.
2. Add the broth and cook for 2 to 3 minutes so the onion absorbs the flavor.
3. Add the lentils and stir. Add the turmeric, curry powder, black pepper, and rice, if using.
4. Add 7 cups water and bring to a boil over high heat, then reduce to medium-low heat and cook for 20 to 25 minutes, until the lentils are soft. Serve.

SERVING SUGGESTION: Dr. Khoshaba's favorite way to eat this is with chopped red onions and a bit of sriracha sauce on top; add ½ serving of protein for a complete meal

GLUTEN-FREE OPTION: No modification needed

VEGAN OPTION: No modification needed

AIP OPTION: No option

White Bean Chile Verde

People will be blown away when you tell them you made this from scratch! They don't have to know how easy it is to make. Tomatillos are found in most supermarkets today. To find good ones, peel away some of the papery husk and look at the skin. It should be bright green and firm.

SERVES 4 **PREP TIME: 15 MINUTES** **TOTAL TIME: 45 MINUTES**

- 1 pound fresh tomatillos, husks removed and tomatillos rinsed well
- 1 serrano chile, stem removed
- 3 garlic cloves
- 1 medium onion, diced
- 1 pound skinless boneless chicken breast, cut into quarters
- ½ (14.5-ounce) BPA-free, no salt added can white beans, with canning liquid
- 1 tablespoon ground cumin
- ½ teaspoon white pepper
- 3 tablespoons unsalted chicken or vegetable broth
- Juice from 2 limes
- 1 bunch fresh cilantro, coarsely chopped

1. Preheat the oven to 425°F. Line a baking sheet with parchment paper or a silicone mat.
2. Place the tomatillos, chile, garlic, and onion on the baking sheet. Roast on the middle rack of the oven for 15 to 20 minutes, until the tomatillos start to brown.
3. In a large saucepan over low heat, combine the chicken, beans and canning liquid, cumin, white pepper, and broth. Whisk to mix well. Reduce the heat to low and simmer, uncovered, for 5 minutes.
4. Place the roasted vegetables in a blender and add 2 cups water. Cover loosely so some steam can escape and blend until almost completely pureed, leaving some small chunks, 60 to 90 seconds.
5. Add the puree to the saucepan, then continue simmering for 25 minutes more. Stir in the lime juice and cilantro just before serving.

GLUTEN-FREE OPTION: No modification needed
VEGAN OPTION: Omit the chicken and use vegetable-flavored bouillon
AIP OPTION: Replace the beans with cauliflower

Homestyle Beef Stew

It has taken many years for me to make a stew that Kirin loves. The ones I used to make were complicated Irish versions that included over a dozen ingredients. This is a great example of how fewer ingredients sometimes lead to cleaner flavors. If you read the recipe and think I forgot to include liquid, know that I did not. You don't have to use a drop, because the ingredients themselves have plenty of moisture to give. Use a heavy pot with a tight-fitting lid. Pressure cookers also work well for this recipe. Potato flesh is low in iodine, but the skins may carry moderate amounts, so it's best to peel.

SERVES 4   **PREP TIME: 5 MINUTES**   **TOTAL TIME: 1 HOUR, 40 MINUTES**

- Avocado oil in a mister or nonstick cooking spray
- 1 pound boneless extra-lean beef stew meat
- 1 medium yellow or sweet onion, diced
- 3 medium Yukon Gold potatoes, peeled and quartered
- 8 ounces baby carrots, cut in half
- 3 celery stalks, sliced
- ¼ cup unsalted beef or vegetable broth

1. Heat a Dutch oven or large, heavy pot over high heat. Mist with the avocado oil. Add the meat and sear, turning to brown on all sides, about 10 minutes.
2. Add the onion and sauté until soft, about 4 minutes.
3. Add the potatoes, carrots, celery, and broth. Cover tightly and reduce the heat to low. Simmer 80 to 90 minutes, or until the meat is tender. Serve.

GLUTEN-FREE OPTION: No modification needed

VEGAN OPTION: Omit the meat or replace with cubed meat substitute or other vegatable protein

AIP OPTION: Omit the potatoes or replace them with cauliflower; add a side of carbs

15-Bean Soup

Okay, maybe it is 13 or 17, but it is easy to find bags of combined dried beans. This is one of the few cases when I suggest soaking your beans ahead. The reason is that these combo packages contain beans that range greatly in size and therefore in their cooking times. By soaking them first, they end up closer to evenly cooked. This is a good dish to put in the slow cooker and forget about until later.

SERVES 8 **PREP TIME: 15 MINUTES, PLUS 8 TO 24 HOURS SOAKING** **TOTAL TIME: 2 HOURS**

- 1 (1-pound) bag 15-bean soup mix
- Avocado oil in a mister or nonstick cooking spray
- 1 medium onion, diced
- 2 garlic cloves, minced
- 2 medium carrots, peeled and sliced
- 2 celery stalks, sliced
- 1 (15-ounce) BPA-free can unsalted diced tomatoes
- 1 teaspoon dried oregano
- 1 teaspoon ground cumin
- 2 teaspoons smoked paprika
- 1 teaspoon cayenne pepper

1. Rinse the beans and place in a large bowl. Cover with about 10 cups water and soak for 8 to 24 hours.
2. Drain the beans and place in a stockpot. Add 8 cups water and bring to a simmer. Cook until the beans are almost tender, about 60 minutes.
3. Mist a large skillet with the avocado oil and heat over medium-high heat. Add the onion, garlic, carrots, celery, tomatoes, oregano, cumin, paprika, and cayenne and sauté for 3 to 4 minutes, until the carrots and celery are tender.
4. Add the vegetables to the pot and simmer an additional 30 minutes, or until the largest beans are soft.

SERVING SUGGESTION: Serve with basic greens and protein for a simple dinner
GLUTEN-FREE OPTION: No modification needed
VEGAN OPTION: No modification needed
AIP OPTION: No option available

Soup of the Green Goddess

Talk about getting your greens. This soup is excellent and ridiculously good for you. Just don't wear a white shirt when you eat it.

SERVES 6   PREP TIME: **10 MINUTES**   TOTAL TIME: **30 MINUTES**

- 2 cups frozen peas
- 3 cups spinach leaves
- 2 cups kale leaves, ribs and thick stems removed
- ½ cup fresh mint leaves
- ½ cup fresh cilantro leaves
- 1 avocado
- ¼ cup unsalted vegetable broth
- Salt and freshly ground black pepper
- 1 cup unflavored non-dairy yogurt
- Avocado oil in a mister or nonstick cooking spray
- 1 medium yellow or sweet onion, diced

1. In a blender, combine the peas, spinach, kale, mint, cilantro, avocado, broth, 2 cups water, salt and pepper, and non-dairy yogurt. Blend well, working in batches if needed, until smooth.

2. Mist a large stockpot with the avocado oil and heat over medium heat. Add the onion and sauté for 2 minutes or until translucent.

3. Add the vegetable puree to the sautéed corn and bring to a simmer, then reduce the heat to low and simmer for 20 minutes. Serve.

SERVING SUGGESTION: Serve with a side of protein for a complete meal
GLUTEN-FREE OPTION: No modification needed
VEGAN OPTION: No modification needed
AIP OPTION: No modification needed

Classic Split Pea Soup

This is always one of my family's favorite comfort meals. You can include leftover meat, add veggie protein, or leave it as is. I like the soup thick, but if you prefer a thinner consistency, add 1 to 2 more cups of water. If you want to use whole dried peas, add an extra cup of water and allow an extra hour to cook.

SERVES 8 PREP TIME: 10 MINUTES TOTAL TIME: 1 HOUR, 35 MINUTES

- Avocado oil in a mister or nonstick cooking spray
- 1 medium yellow or sweet onion, diced
- 2 cups green split peas
- 3 celery stalks with leaves, chopped
- 3 medium carrots, chopped
- ¼ cup unsalted vegetable broth
- Salt and freshly ground black pepper

1. Mist a large stockpot with the avocado oil and heat over medium heat. Add the onion and sauté for 2 minutes or until translucent.
2. Add the peas, celery, and carrots and sauté an additional 3 minutes.
3. Add the broth, 7 cups water, and salt and pepper and bring to boil. Reduce the heat to low and simmer about 90 minutes, until the peas are tender and the vegetables are cooked.

SERVING SUGGESTION: Add protein for a complete meal; you can also include additional greens

GLUTEN-FREE OPTION: No modification needed

VEGAN OPTION: No modification needed

AIP OPTION: For peas, substitute 2 pounds of asparagus, steamed and pureed, and 2 diced medium avocados; reduce the liquid to 2 cups water and reduce the cooking time to 15 minutes; add a carb and a protein

Curried Kabocha Soup

Kabocha is a winter squash, also called a Japanese pumpkin. The flavor is more pronounced and earthy than other winter squashes. If you can't find kabocha, butternut or acorn squash can be used in the same way. And don't waste the seeds! You can clean off the filaments, rinse, and toast them in a 250°F oven for about 20 minutes. They can then be sprinkled on the soup or served separately as a snack. Count them toward your healthy fat intake.

SERVES 6 **PREP TIME: 10 MINUTES** **TOTAL TIME: 30 MINUTES**

- 1 (2- to 3-pound) kabocha squash, seeded and sliced into quarters
- 1 yellow or sweet onion, diced
- 1 (2-inch) piece fresh ginger, sliced
- 4 cups unsalted vegetable broth
- ¾ cup unsweetened non-dairy milk (flax or coconut milk work well)
- 2 tablespoons red curry paste

1. Preheat the oven to 350°F. Line a baking sheet with parchment paper or a silicone mat.
2. Place the squash pieces on the baking sheet, cut side up. Sprinkle the onion and ginger on top. Bake about 50 minutes, until the squash is fork-tender.
3. Let cool, then scoop the squash flesh free of the peel and discard the peel.
4. In a blender, combine the squash, onion, and ginger with the broth, non-dairy milk, and curry paste. Blend, loosely covered, for 2 minutes, until smooth.
5. Serve immediately or refrigerate for a later meal.

GLUTEN-FREE OPTION: No modification needed
VEGAN OPTION: No modification needed
AIP OPTION: Omit non-dairy beverage

Calamari Stew

If you like tomato-based seafood stews, here is an excellent low-iodine option.

SERVES 4 **PREP TIME: 15 MINUTES** **TOTAL TIME: 75 MINUTES**

- Avocado oil in a mister or nonstick cooking spray
- 1 medium onion, diced
- 1 fennel bulb and fronds, outer tough leaves removed, bulb chopped
- 2 tablespoons unsalted tomato paste
- ¼ cup white wine vinegar
- 3 garlic cloves, minced
- 2 pounds calamari (squid), chopped
- 1 (28-ounce) BPA-free can unsalted crushed tomatoes
- 1 tablespoon extra-virgin olive oil
- Salt and freshly ground black pepper
- ½ cup chopped fresh parsley

1. Mist a large skillet with the avocado oil and heat over medium-high heat until hot enough to sizzle a drop of water. Add the onion and fennel and sauté about 3 minutes, until the onion is translucent.

2. Add the tomato paste, vinegar, and garlic and sauté an additional 3 minutes or until the sauce is reduced to one-fourth the amount you started with. Stir frequently so the garlic doesn't burn.

3. Add the calamari and crushed tomatoes and lower the heat to medium low. Simmer for 5 to 10 minutes, or until the calamari is tender; don't overcook.

4. Season with salt and pepper and garnish with the parsley.

SERVING SUGGESTION: Serve with a good carb for a complete meal

GLUTEN-FREE OPTION: No modification needed

VEGAN OPTION: Replace the squid with seitan and increase the final simmer time from 10 minutes to 45 minutes

AIP OPTION: No option available

MAIN COURSES

Homestyle Meatloaf

Any kind of ground meat can work well in this meatloaf. I use 93 percent lean ground beef or ground turkey. One tip for a nice texture is to not mix it too vigorously. Once the ingredients are (mostly) evenly distributed, it is time for it to go into the pan. Also, an easy way to puree the beans is to pour off just a bit of the liquid and insert an immersion blender right into the can!

SERVES 4 **PREP TIME: 10 MINUTES** **TOTAL TIME: 1 HOUR, 10 MINUTES**

- 1 (14.5-ounce) BPA-free, no salt added can black beans
- Avocado oil in a mister or nonstick cooking spray
- 1 medium yellow or sweet onion, diced
- 4 ounces fresh button mushrooms, finely chopped
- 1 pound 93 percent lean ground beef or ground turkey
- 1 green bell pepper, cored, seeded, and diced
- 3 garlic cloves, minced
- ½ cup liquid egg whites
- 1 teaspoon dried thyme
- 1 teaspoon dried parsley
- 1 teaspoon salt
- ½ teaspoon freshly ground black pepper
- 1 tablespoon unsalted tomato paste

1. Preheat the oven to 400°F.
2. Drain the beans and reserve half the canning liquid. Puree the beans and remaining canning liquid in a food processor or use an immersion blender right in the can.
3. Mist a large skillet with the avocado oil, then heat over medium-high heat until hot enough to sizzle a drop of water.

4. Add the onion and mushrooms and sauté for 2 to 3 minutes, until onion is translucent.

5. Place the onion and mushrooms in a large bowl and add the meat, bean puree, bell pepper, garlic, egg whites, thyme, parsley, salt, pepper, and tomato paste. Stir to blend the ingredients, then shape into a loaf.

6. Mist an 8 by 4 by 2½-inch loaf pan with some avocado oil, then transfer the loaf to the pan, cover with aluminum foil, and bake for 1 hour, or until the internal temperature reaches 160°F. Let rest briefly, then serve or refrigerate for later use.

SERVING SUGGESTION: Serve with a side of greens and a good carb for a complete meal

GLUTEN-FREE OPTION: No modification needed

VEGAN OPTION: Use ground meat substitute and omit the egg whites; instead, add ½ cup old-fashioned rolled oats

AIP OPTION: Omit the tomato paste

Shepherd's Pie

This is an update on the all-time favorite comfort food recipe from *The Adrenal Reset Diet*. I've made this with vegan ground "meat," and it worked perfectly. Just be sure to avoid any products made with seaweed-based binders (carrageenan, alginates, agar-agar).

SERVES 4 **PREP TIME: 40 MINUTES** **TOTAL TIME: 1 HOUR, 20 MINUTES**

- 1 tablespoon salt
- 3 cups peeled and diced russet potatoes (from 3 to 4 potatoes)
- Avocado oil in a mister or nonstick cooking spray
- 8 ounces lean ground meat substitute
- 1 medium yellow or sweet onion, diced
- 8 ounces fresh button mushrooms, sliced
- 3 medium carrots, sliced into thin coins
- 2 celery stalks, chopped
- 3 tablespoons unsalted beef or vegetable broth

1. Preheat the oven to 350°F.
2. Bring a large pot of water to a boil and add the salt. Add the potatoes, reduce the heat to medium, and simmer for 12 minutes, or until the potatoes split easily with a fork. Drain and mash the potatoes with a potato masher or in a food processor; add a little cooking water or broth to soften, if necessary.
3. Mist a large skillet with the avocado oil and heat on medium-high heat until a drop of water sizzles. Add the meat and brown it, stirring, for 4 to 5 minutes. Transfer to a plate.
4. Add the onion to the skillet and sauté until translucent, about 2 minutes.
5. Add the mushrooms and sauté until soft, 1 to 2 minutes. Then add the carrots, celery, and broth. Stir and sauté for 3 minutes, then add the meat, and stir to combine.
6. Pour the meat mixture into a 2-quart casserole dish and spread the mashed potatoes evenly over the top. Cover with aluminum foil and bake for 25 minutes. Then uncover and bake an additional 10 minutes, until potato topping is lightly browned in spots.

SERVING SUGGESTION: This can be a one-course meal or serve it with cooked greens
GLUTEN-FREE OPTION: No modification needed
VEGAN OPTION: Replace the meat with ground meat substitute
AIP OPTION: Replace the potatoes with cooked and mashed cauliflower florets

Minnesota-Style Wild Rice Hot Dish

This was my favorite dish growing up. At every major family get-together, at least one person always made some version of this casserole. Cream of mushroom soup was the staple thickener, but it has too much fat and poor-quality ingredients. After many attempts, I've improved it with healthy ingredients. All types of wild rice are good, but most are farm-grown in California. Those have narrow, black grains, but the real Minnesota lake rice has larger and less narrow grains. They are also a flecked light tan, almost white and black. If you can get the real thing, you'll have a special treat. The overnight soak is helpful so that the rice cooks completely. This also makes excellent leftovers!

SERVES 6

PREP TIME: 20 MINUTES, PLUS OVERNIGHT SOAK

TOTAL TIME: 1 HOUR, 20 MINUTES

- 1 cup wild rice
- 1 cup long-grain brown rice
- 1 pound 93 percent lean ground beef or turkey
- 2 tablespoons arrowroot powder
- 2 cups unsalted vegetable broth
- 8 ounces fresh medium mushrooms (such as whitecap), sliced
- 2 cups unflavored non-dairy milk (such as unsweetened flax milk)
- 1 medium yellow or sweet onion, diced
- 1 pound frozen French-cut green beans
- 3 celery stalks with leaves, chopped
- 3 garlic cloves, minced

1. Combine the wild and brown rices in a large bowl. Cover with 3 inches of water and let soak overnight at room temperature. Drain and rinse the rice.
2. Preheat the oven to 400°F.
3. In a large skillet over medium heat, brown the meat for 3 to 5 minutes. Transfer to a large bowl.

4. Mix the arrowroot with the broth. Add to the bowl along with the rice, mushrooms, non-dairy milk, onion, beans, celery, and garlic. Stir well to mix all ingredients.

5. Pour the mixture into a 9 by 13-inch baking pan and cover with a lid or aluminum foil. Bake for 60 minutes, or until bubbly. Let rest for 10 minutes, then serve.

SERVING SUGGESTION: Serve with additional vegetables

GLUTEN-FREE OPTION: No modification needed

VEGAN OPTION: Omit the ground meat or replace with 1 (12-ounce) package tempeh, crumbled and browned

AIP OPTION: If in the reintroduction stage, omit the brown rice and replace with an additional cup of wild rice

Paprika Chicken with Roasted Limas and Brussels Sprouts

This is an unusual dish that is exotic enough for entertaining, yet surprisingly easy to prepare.

SERVES 4   PREP TIME: **20 MINUTES**   TOTAL TIME: **1 HOUR**

- 2 pounds skin-on, bone-in chicken breasts
- 2 tablespoons olive oil
- Spice blend of choice
- 1 (14.5-ounce) BPA-free, no salt added can lima beans, drained
- 1 pound Brussels sprouts, trimmed and cut in half lengthwise
- 1 cup red seedless grapes
- 2 teaspoons smoked paprika
- 2 teaspoons ground cumin
- 1 teaspoon dried garlic
- 1 teaspoon salt

1. Preheat the oven to 400°F. Line a rimmed baking sheet (sheet pan) with parchment paper or a silicone mat.
2. In a large bowl, coat the chicken breasts with 1 tablespoon of the olive oil and half the spice blend.
3. Place the chicken on the baking sheet and roast on the middle rack of the oven for 15 minutes.
4. In a medium bowl, combine the lima beans, sprouts, grapes, paprika, cumin, garlic, salt, the remaining olive oil, and the remaining spice blend.
5. Spoon the vegetable mixture around the chicken breasts and return to the oven to roast roughly 35 minutes more, or until the sprouts are lightly browned and fork-tender. The chicken should register 165°F on an instant-read thermometer. Let rest 5 minutes, then serve as a complete meal.

GLUTEN-FREE OPTION: No modification needed
VEGAN OPTION: Omit the chicken or replace with 1½ pounds of cubed tempeh
AIP OPTION: Omit the lima beans

Creamy Tarragon Chicken

When you taste this chicken, you'll be amazed it is dairy-free. Potatoes give the dish its texture, as well as a whole new level of satisfaction. This is a wonderful comfort meal. Unfortunately, I had to forgo the potato peels, as some studies have shown they can be high in iodine.

SERVES 4 **PREP TIME: 25 MINUTES** **TOTAL TIME: 65 MINUTES**

- 3 to 4 Yukon Gold potatoes (1½ pounds), peeled
- Avocado oil in a mister or nonstick cooking spray
- 4 skinless boneless chicken tenders (roughly 2 pounds)
- ¼ cup white wine vinegar
- ½ yellow or sweet onion, diced
- 8 ounces fresh button mushrooms, sliced
- 2 garlic cloves, crushed
- 1 pound frozen green beans
- 3 tablespoons unsalted chicken broth
- 1 teaspoon dried tarragon
- 1 tablespoon olive oil

1. In a medium saucepan, cover the potatoes in water and boil for 12 minutes or until easily split with a fork. Drain the potatoes and reserve 2 cups of the cooking water. Allow the potatoes to cool for 10 minutes.

2. In a blender, combine the potatoes and cooking water. Open the blender vent slightly so steam can escape.

3. Mist a large skillet with the avocado oil and heat on medium-high heat until a drop of water sizzles.

4. Place the chicken in the skillet and cook for 4 minutes, then turn and cook an additional 2 minutes or until cooked through. Transfer the chicken to a plate, cover, and keep warm.

5. Add the vinegar to the skillet, then add the onion and simmer it for 3 minutes, until translucent. Add the mushrooms and garlic and sauté for 2 to 3 minutes, until the mushrooms are softened. Be careful not to burn the garlic.

6. Stir in the broth, tarragon, green beans, and blended potatoes. Cover and simmer for 15 minutes.

7. Spread the bean mixture on 4 serving plates and top with the chicken.

SERVE AS A COMPLETE MEAL

GLUTEN-FREE OPTION: No modification needed

VEGAN OPTION: Omit the chicken or substitute seitan or tempeh; use vegetable broth instead of chicken broth

AIP OPTION: Substitute acorn squash for the potato

Gingered Tempeh and Broccoli

Tempeh is a traditional fermented soy food first used in Indonesian cuisine. It is a complete protein and is rich in fiber, micronutrients, prebiotics, and antioxidants. Most large health food supermarkets carry it in the refrigerated or frozen food section.

SERVES 4 **PREP TIME: 10 MINUTES** **TOTAL TIME: 20 MINUTES**

- 1 tablespoon avocado oil
- 2 (12-ounce) packages tempeh (or 3 [8-ounce] packages), thawed and cut into bite-size pieces
- 2 fresh lemongrass stalks, roots and outer leaves discarded, white section finely chopped; or 2 tablespoons dried lemongrass
- 2 garlic cloves, minced
- 1 head of broccoli, cut into florets
- 1 pound green beans, cut into 2-inch sections
- 1 medium onion, sliced
- 1 tablespoon honey
- ½ to 1 teaspoon red pepper flakes
- 2 tablespoons tamari

1. Place the oil in a wok or large skillet and put over medium-high heat; heat until a drop of water sizzles.
2. Add the tempeh and stir-fry for 3 to 5 minutes, until it starts to brown.
3. Add the lemongrass and garlic, and stir-fry an additional 2 minutes.
4. Add ½ cup water along with the broccoli, green beans, onion, honey, red pepper flakes, and tamari. Stir-fry an additional 5 minutes or until the vegetables are cooked and colorful. Serve.

SERVING SUGGESTION: Serve this over steamed brown rice

GLUTEN-FREE OPTION: No modification needed

VEGAN OPTION: No modification needed

AIP OPTION: Substitute coconut aminos for the tamari, and serve over riced cauliflower

Kirin's Slow-Cooker Chicken

This is a two-ingredient recipe (plus oil and salt and pepper) that will amaze people! You can set the flavor based on the herbs or seasonings you add. We keep it simple and use just a bit of salt and pepper. This simple preparation allows you to use the leftovers in soups and salads. You don't need any liquid for this because the onion gives it just enough moisture to make this juicy and fall-off-the-bone delicious.

SERVES 4 TO 6   PREP TIME: 5 MINUTES   TOTAL TIME: 4 HOURS

- Avocado oil in a mister or nonstick cooking spray
- 1 large yellow or sweet onion, sliced (6 to 8 slices)
- 1 (3- to 4-pound) chicken, rinsed and patted dry
- Salt and freshly ground black pepper

1. Set the slow cooker on high heat and let it heat up for 5 minutes.
2. Mist the liner pot with a little avocado oil, then lay the onion slices in the liner pot so they cover the bottom. Place the chicken on top of the onion slices, breast side down.
3. Cover with the lid, and turn the heat to low. Let cook for 4 hours, or until the chicken legs wiggle freely and the breasts give with with light pressure.
4. Remove from cooker and lightly dust with salt and pepper.

SERVING SUGGESTION: Serve with veggies and a good carb, such as cooked spinach and brown rice

GLUTEN-FREE OPTION: No modification needed

VEGAN OPTION: No option available

AIP OPTION: No modification needed

One-Pot Green Chile Pasta

This is one of my wife, Kirin's, favorites! If you've never made a one-pot pasta dish, you're in for a treat.

SERVES 4 **PREP TIME: 10 MINUTES** **TOTAL TIME: 25 MINUTES**

- Avocado oil in a mister or nonstick cooking spray
- 1 pound lean ground turkey
- Salt and freshly ground black pepper
- 3 teaspoons ground cumin
- 1 teaspoon dried oregano
- ¼ teaspoon cayenne pepper
- 4 garlic cloves, minced
- 1 medium yellow or sweet onion, diced
- 1 red bell pepper, cored, seeded, and diced
- 1 (4-ounce) can Hatch green chiles or other canned green chiles
- 1 (10-ounce) can unsalted diced tomatoes
- 1 (12-ounce) box whole-grain penne pasta
- 2 tablespoons unsalted chicken or vegetable broth
- ¼ cup unflavored non-dairy milk
- 3 cups fresh spinach leaves
- 1 bunch fresh cilantro, chopped

1. Mist a large, heavy saucepan with the avocado oil. Heat over medium-high heat until a drop of water sizzles.

2. Add the turkey and brown for 3 to 5 minutes, until cooked through.

3. Season the turkey with salt and pepper. Add the cumin, oregano, and cayenne. Stir well and cook for 1 minute, then add the garlic, onion, and bell pepper. Cook an additional 3 minutes, until vegetables are softened.

4. Pour in the chiles and tomatoes. Add the pasta, chicken broth, and 2 cups water. Cover, reduce the heat to medium low, and simmer for 7 to 9 minutes, as per pasta cooking time.

5. Uncover, add the non-dairy milk and spinach, and stir for about 3 minutes, until the spinach is wilted. Transfer to serving plates and garnish with the cilantro.

SERVE AS A COMPLETE MEAL

GLUTEN-FREE OPTION: Use gluten-free penne pasta

VEGAN OPTION: Use 2 cups of cooked lentils in place of the turkey

AIP OPTION: Use cooked spaghetti squash or zucchini noodles in place of the pasta, and omit the tomatoes and cayenne

Chicken with Peaches and Black Beans

If you're in a rush, you can blend the veggies in a food processor or small blender until it's in salsa-size bits. Adjust the jalapeños per your spice tolerance. And be sure to wear gloves or at least wash your hands twice after handling the chiles!

SERVES 4   PREP TIME: 10 MINUTES   TOTAL TIME: 35 MINUTES

- Avocado oil in a mister or nonstick cooking spray
- 1 pound skinless boneless chicken breasts, cubed
- 2 peaches, pits removed, diced in ½-inch pieces
- 2 Roma (plum) tomatoes, diced in ½-inch pieces
- 1 medium onion, finely diced
- 2 jalapeño peppers, seeded and finely diced
- 1 avocado, diced in ½-inch pieces
- 1 (15-ounce) BPA-free can, no salt added black beans, drained and rinsed
- Salt and freshly ground black pepper
- ½ bunch fresh cilantro, chopped

1. Mist a large skillet with the avocado oil. Heat the skillet over high heat until hot enough that a drop of water sizzles.
2. Add the chicken, stir, and sauté for 5 minutes or until just cooked.
3. Add the peaches, tomatoes, onion, jalapeños, avocado, and beans. Stir for an additional minute, until warmed through.
4. Season with salt and pepper, and garnish with the cilantro.

SERVING SUGGESTION: Add a side of mixed vegetables
GLUTEN-FREE OPTION: No modification needed
VEGAN OPTION: Omit the chicken or replace with cooked seitan
AIP OPTION: Omit the beans and tomatoes or replace with a cubed roasted sweet potato

Creamy Lentil Curry

You'll be amazed at what a perfect "cream" a mashed potato can make. For dishes like these, russets work nicely for texture, but red potatoes are the next best option. Fun fact: red lentils are the same as green or brown lentils—just without the skin.

SERVES 4 TO 6 **PREP TIME: 10 MINUTES** **TOTAL TIME: 30 MINUTES**

- Avocado oil in a mister or nonstick cooking spray
- 1 medium yellow or sweet onion, diced
- 2 tablespoons curry powder
- 1 tablespoon nutritional yeast
- 1 teaspoon ground turmeric, or 2 teaspoons grated fresh turmeric
- 1 tablespoon unsalted vegetable bouillon powder
- 3 cups diced peeled russet potatoes (from 3 to 4 medium potatoes)
- 2 cups red lentils, rinsed and drained
- 3 medium carrots, sliced
- 2 celery stalks, chopped
- 3 cups chopped fresh kale

1. Mist a large, heavy saucepan with avocado oil. Heat the saucepan over medium-high heat until a drop of water sizzles.
2. Add the onion and sauté for 3 minutes, until translucent.
3. Stir in the curry powder, yeast, turmeric, and bouillon powder and stir another 1 minute.
4. Add the potatoes, lentils, carrots, celery, and 6 cups water. Reduce the heat to medium low and simmer for 25 minutes, or until the potatoes are soft.
5. Add the kale and simmer an additional 2 minutes, until the kale is wilted.
6. Remove 1 to 1½ cups of the mixture along with 2 cups of the liquid and place in a blender and blend until smooth, with the vent slightly open so steam can escape (blend in batches, if necessary).
7. Add the puree to the saucepan and stir until well incorporated. Serve.

SERVING SUGGESTION: Though lentils are higher in protein than other legumes, they are not quite high enough for this to be a full serving of protein; accompany with ½ serving of protein

GLUTEN-FREE OPTION: No modification needed

VEGAN OPTION: No modification needed

AIP OPTION: Replace the lentils with any cooked meat; replace the potatoes with cauliflower florets and reduce the cooking to 15 minutes

Poached Garlic Chicken

Is your family bored with chicken? Here is an easy brined chicken recipe that will make everyone see the bird in a new light. Also, leaner cuts of poultry, in general, often cook up dry and flavorless, but brining yields a moist result. A kitchen thermometer is helpful for the best results. I like to serve this poached chicken with mildly flavored side dishes so the chicken's full flavor gets a chance to shine for a change.

SERVES 4 TO 6   PREP TIME: **10 MINUTES**   TOTAL TIME: **1 HOUR, 55 MINUTES**

- 1 tablespoon honey
- ½ cup tamari
- ¼ cup kosher salt (for brining)
- 1 large head of garlic, cloves separated, larger cloves mashed
- 4 (6- to 8-ounce) skinless boneless chicken breasts

1. In a large pot, whisk together the honey, tamari, salt, garlic, and 4 quarts water. Add the chicken breasts and let sit at room temperature for 30 minutes.
2. Place the pot on the stove over low heat so the temperature in the pot rises to 175°F; check with a thermometer. Allow 25 to 35 minutes.
3. Simmer the chicken at this temperature for 20 minutes, then turn off the heat and cover the pot. Let sit for an additional 20 minutes, then remove from the pot and discard the water. Serve the chicken.

SERVING SUGGESTION: Serve with a side of vegetables and good carbs, such as greens, alliums, and cruciferous veggies (see page 234), as well as steamed millet
GLUTEN-FREE OPTION: No modification needed
VEGAN OPTION: No option available
AIP OPTION: No modification needed

Better Than Carry-Out Orange Chicken

Orange chicken was my son's go-to dish whenever it was on the menu at a Chinese restaurant. He never had it more than a couple of times per year, but every so often I tried to win him over with a homemade version. He was polite about my many versions, but this was the first one that he preferred over the restaurants'. Instead of the fresh orange zest, organic dried orange peel works well, but then you need only 2 tablespoons.

SERVES 4 **PREP TIME: 15 MINUTES** **TOTAL TIME: 45 MINUTES**

- ¼ cup freshly grated orange zest
- Juice from 2 oranges (roughly ⅔ cup)
- 1 tablespoon honey
- 2 garlic cloves, crushed
- 1 tablespoon grated fresh ginger
- ¼ cup tamari
- 2 tablespoons dry sherry
- ½ teaspoon toasted sesame oil
- 2 tablespoons arrowroot powder
- 1 pound skinless boneless chicken breasts, cut into bite-sized pieces
- Salt and freshly ground black pepper
- Avocado oil in a mister or nonstick cooking spray
- 1 bunch scallions, trimmed, sliced lengthwise into quarters, then cut into 1-inch pieces
- 1 red bell pepper, cored, seeded, and sliced into matchstick strips

1. In a small saucepan, combine the orange zest, orange juice, honey, garlic, ginger, tamari, sherry, and sesame oil. Dissolve the arrowroot powder in ½ cup water, then add to the saucepan. Simmer over low heat for 10 minutes. Set aside.

2. Season the chicken with salt and pepper and let sit at room temperature for 10 minutes.

3. Mist a large skillet or wok with the avocado oil. Heat over medium-high heat until a drop of water sizzles. Add the chicken and stir-fry for 5 to 7 minutes, until just cooked. Transfer to a plate.

4. Add the scallions and red pepper to the skillet and stir-fry for 1 to 2 minutes, until the peppers becomes brighter in color.

5. Add the chicken and sauce to the skillet and briefly stir. Simmer for 2 to 3 minutes, then serve.

SERVING SUGGESTION: Serve over cooked brown rice and add a side of vegetables
GLUTEN-FREE OPTION: No modification needed
VEGAN OPTION: Use cooked seitan, cut into bite-size pieces, in place of the chicken
AIP OPTION: Omit the sherry, substitute coconut aminos for the tamari, and serve over riced cauliflower

Cajun Catfish

Catfish has gotten a bad rap, owing to the omega 6 content and the fact that the fish is a scavenger. Too much of any food constituent is harmful, but all foods with fat have a combination of types of fat; for example, 1 tablespoon of olive oil contains about 1,300 mg of omega 6 fat. A 3-ounce serving of catfish has about 131 mg of omega 6. As for being a scavenger, most catfish sold in the U.S. markets are farm-raised in America. Some wild catfish from Asia and Europe can be high in toxic metals, but it is not commonly available here. Actually, catfish is among the fish that are lowest in mercury and other toxins, so it is considered one of the safest to eat. It is a rich source of vitamin B12, magnesium, zinc, and more. Thankfully, it is also a low-iodine fish.

SERVES 4 **PREP TIME: 20 MINUTES** **TOTAL TIME: 30 MINUTES**

- 1 teaspoon salt
- 1 teaspoon freshly ground black pepper
- 1 teaspoon garlic powder
- 1 teaspoon onion powder
- 1 teaspoon smoked paprika
- 1 teaspoon dried parsley
- 1 teaspoon cayenne pepper
- ½ teaspoon dried oregano
- ½ teaspoon dried thyme
- 1 pound catfish fillets
- Avocado oil in a mister or nonstick cooking spray

1. Mix the salt, pepper, garlic and onion powder, paprika, parsley, cayenne, oregano, and thyme in a shallow bowl or on a sheet of wax paper.
2. Lay the catfish fillets in the spice mixture, turning to coat each side.
3. Mist a large skillet with the avocado oil and heat over medium-high heat until a drop of oil sizzles in the pan.
4. Place the catfish in the skillet, working in 2 batches if necessary. Sauté for 2 minutes, then turn and cook on the other side for approximately 1 minute, or until the flesh just starts to flake and the fillets are lightly browned. Serve.

SERVING SUGGESTION: Serve with a side of good carbs and vegetables

GLUTEN-FREE OPTION: No modification needed

VEGAN OPTION: Substitute firm tofu; rinse and slice into ½-inch-thick rectangles, then place between layers of dish towel and place a weight on top; press for 20 minutes, then use it in place of the catfish

AIP OPTION: Omit the black pepper, cayenne, and paprika

Garlic-Lime Calamari

Calamari (squid) is among the most sustainable seafood available. It is easy to find, low in cost, low in iodine, and super easy to work with in the kitchen. You can buy a whole squid or portions. Many supermarkets have it frozen and those with large seafood departments will have it fresh. Calamari steaks and tubes are interchangeable; if you cut a tube lengthwise, you've got a steak. I've made calamari multiple times in different ways, but this is by far my biggest hit.

SERVES 4   **PREP TIME: 5 MINUTES**   **TOTAL TIME: 15 MINUTES**

- Avocado oil in a mister or nonstick cooking spray
- 1 pound fresh or thawed calamari, rinsed and patted dry
- 2 tablespoons neutral oil, such as avocado oil
- 4 garlic cloves, minced
- ½ cup white wine vinegar
- 1 lime, quartered

1. Mist a large skillet with the avocado oil and heat over medium-high heat until a drop of water sizzles.
2. Add the calamari, leaving 1 inch or more between each piece; cook in batches, if necessary. (If cooking in batches, cool and wipe the pan clean pan between batches.) Lightly mist the calamari with some oil and cook for 2 to 3 minutes. Turn and cook for another 2 to 3 minutes, until the flesh is just firm. Transfer to serving plates and keep warm.
3. Heat a medium skillet over medium heat. Add the avocado oil and the garlic. Cook 2 to 3 minutes, until transparent. Add the vinegar and stir frequently until reduced by half, usually 3 to 5 minutes.
4. Squeeze the lime juice into the vinegar and stir for another minute.
5. Pour the sauce over the calamari and serve immediately.

SERVING SUGGESTION: Serve with a side of good carbs and vegetables

GLUTEN-FREE OPTION: No modification needed

VEGAN OPTION: Use firm tofu in place of the calamari; rinse and slice into ½-inch-thick rectangles, place between layers of a dish towel and place a weight on top, and press for 20 minutes, then cook as for the calamari.

AIP OPTION: Omit the garlic and vinegar

Chermoula Baked River Trout

Chermoula is a Moroccan sauce that usually includes cilantro, paprika, cumin, and garlic. This flavor combination works well with a light fish like river trout, which is lower in iodine than other seafood.

SERVES 4   **PREP TIME: 5 MINUTES**   **TOTAL TIME: 25 MINUTES**

- 1 pound fresh or thawed previously frozen river trout fillets
- 1 fresh lemon, sliced
- ¼ cup chopped fresh cilantro
- 1 teaspoon paprika
- 3 garlic cloves, crushed
- ½ teaspoon ground cumin
- Salt and freshly ground black pepper

1. Preheat the oven to 350°F. Line a baking sheet with parchment paper.
2. Place the fillets on the baking sheet and sprinkle the lemon slices, cilantro, paprika, garlic, and cumin over the fish. Season with salt and pepper.
3. Bake for 10 to 13 minutes, or until the fish is just starting to flake.
4. Remove the lemon slices and serve.

SERVING SUGGESTION: Serve with a good carb and a side of vegetables

GLUTEN-FREE OPTION: No modification needed

VEGAN OPTION: No option

AIP OPTION: Omit paprika

SIDES, DRESSINGS, AND DIPS

Some of the main dishes are stand-alone meals and some are not. For those that are not, here are some side-dish options to make your meals complete. They can also be handy if you find yourself coming to the end of the day without having had enough of your veggies.

Easy Flatbread

If you miss bread, please know that homemade baked goods are already low in iodine or can easily be adapted. I think this is one of the easiest to make. It is a great accompaniment to a meal or you can use it in wraps and sandwiches.

If you have a scale, it is easier and more accurate to weigh flour instead of measuring it by volume. I like to use some white whole wheat flour instead of all-purpose flour alone. White whole wheat flour is whole wheat flour, but made from a naturally white wheat berry.

MAKES 12 FLATBREADS **PREP TIME: 15 MINUTES** **TOTAL TIME: 1 HOUR**

- 2 cups all-purpose flour (240 grams), plus more for rolling
- 1 cup white whole wheat flour (120 grams)
- 2 teaspoons baking powder
- 1½ teaspoons salt
- 2 tablespoons vegetable oil (avocado, grapeseed, or canola)
- 1 cup ice water
- Nonstick cooking spray

1. In a large bowl, combine the flours, baking powder, and salt. Mix thoroughly with a whisk or a fork.
2. Make a well in the middle of the flour mixture and add the oil and ice water. Gradually bringing the flour into the well, mix until the dough is evenly moistened. Cover with a damp towel and let rest for 10 minutes.
3. Separate the dough into 12 equal pieces. Each will be about the size of a golf ball.

4. On a floured surface, roll out each ball into a round about ¼ inch thick.

5. Heat a large skillet or griddle over medium-high heat and coat with cooking spray.

6. Add the dough rounds to the skillet a few at a time and cook for 2 to 3 minutes on each side or until golden brown.

7. Let cool for 10 minutes before serving. After cooling for 2 to 4 hours, store in an airtight bag with a paper towel or dry dish towel to catch moisture.

GLUTEN-FREE OPTION: Use gluten-free all-purpose flour
VEGAN OPTION: No modification needed
AIP OPTION: No option available

Basic Brown Rice

Here is a good staple to have on hand. Most grains cook by the same procedure, although you may need to adjust the amount of liquid for some.

SERVES 8 **PREP TIME: 5 MINUTES** **TOTAL TIME: 60 MINUTES**

- 2 cups brown rice

1. Rinse the rice with cool water until the water runs clear.
2. Place the rice in a medium saucepan and add 4 cups water. Bring to a rolling boil over high heat, then reduce the heat to low and simmer for 45 minutes covered.
3. Turn off the heat and let rest for 10 minutes before serving.

GLUTEN-FREE OPTION: No modification needed
VEGAN OPTION: No modification needed
AIP OPTION: No option available

Basic Greens

This is my favorite way to prepare greens. A key element is the ume plum vinegar. *Ume* is short for *umeboshi,* a fermented plum used in Japanese cuisine. Most larger health food supermarkets have ume plum vinegar, and you can always find it online.

In this recipe I use baby bok choy, but the preparation works for any type of greens you plan to cook—arugula, beet tops, collards, dandelion, kale, or spinach are all wonderful, too. Do note that cooking times may vary. Collards, kale, and dandelion may take longer, spinach and arugula will need less time.

SERVES 4 **PREP TIME: 4 MINUTES** **TOTAL TIME: 10 MINUTES**

- Avocado oil in a mister or nonstick cooking spray
- 1 bunch bok choy or 4 bunches baby bok choy, white stalks separated from green leaves and chopped into bite-size pieces
- 1 teaspoon sesame seeds
- 2 teaspoons ume plum vinegar

1. Heat a large skillet over medium-high heat and mist with the avocado oil.
2. Add the bok choy stalks and stir continuously for 2 to 3 minutes, until they just start to soften.
3. Add the sesame seeds and bok choy leaves, and stir for another 1 to 2 minutes, or until the leaves wilt. Remove from the heat, stir in ume plum vinegar and serve.

GLUTEN-FREE OPTION: No modification needed
VEGAN OPTION: No modification needed
AIP OPTION: Omit the sesame seeds

Klubb (Norwegian Potato Dumplings)

My family all hunted when I was growing up. I enjoyed our getting together and walking in the cold woods all day, but I never had the heart for shooting deer. Before we went out, Grandma Christianson fed us klubb and packed some for us to take with us. She told us that her klubb would keep us warm and keep us from getting tired. It seemed to work.

Here is a dish I can almost guarantee you've never had before. Consider it one of the best sources of resistant starch! It takes a fair amount of time to drain the potatoes, but the basic idea is to get them as dry as possible. Some recipes omit this step, but the final texture is even heartier when you make that extra effort. The traditional recipe calls for barley flour and whole wheat flour, but you can replace the barley flour with more whole wheat flour. You can also grind pearl barley in a powerful blender to make barley flour.

SERVES 4 OR MORE **PREP TIME: 30 MINUTES** **TOTAL TIME: 2 HOURS**

- 5 large russet potatoes, peeled
- ¾ cup barley flour
- 1 cup whole wheat flour
- 4 teaspoons salt
- Chopped rutabaga, onion, apple, or roast meat (optional)

1. Using a coarse grater, grate the potatoes. If you have a food grinder, you can also use that to grind the potatoes.

2. Place the grated potatoes in a colander in the sink and set a weighted bowl on top to push out the liquid. Let drain for 60 to 90 minutes, then discard the liquid.

3. Place the potatoes in a bowl and mix with the flours and 1 teaspoon salt. Mix to get a thick, dough-like consistency. You may need a bit more or less flour.

4. Bring about 3 quarts of water to a boil in a large saucepan and add the remaining 3 teaspoons salt. Bring to a boil over high heat, then reduce the heat to low.

5. Using an ice-cream scoop or a ⅓ cup measure, scoop up pieces of dough and shape into ovals, then set them on a tray.

6. If desired, push a bite of something tasty into each dumpling. Traditional choices are a piece of rutabaga, onion, apple, or cubes of roasted meat.

7. Using a strainer, lower the dumplings into the water and simmer for 60 minutes.

8. Use the strainer to remove the cooked dumplings and transfer them to serving plates. Serve immediately. (The dumplings can also be refrigerated for up to 5 days or frozen for up to 1 month.)

GLUTEN-FREE OPTION: Use 1½ cups of gluten-free flour instead of the whole wheat and barley flours; Bob's Red Mill gluten-free all-purpose baking flour is my favorite

VEGAN OPTION: No modification needed

AIP OPTION: No option available

Whole-Grain Sourdough Bread

Many of the concerns about commercially baked goods are not inherent in the wheat or other grains but, rather, in the additives that have iodine or a lack of proper fermentation. Commercial bread is made at a rate of hundreds of loaves per minute. There is never time for the yeast and bacteria to predigest the proteins.

You can make sourdough bread with a sourdough starter, or you can use baker's yeast to jump-start the process. But be careful—if you use too much yeast, you will throw off the flavor. Many bread recipes that are meant to rise quickly use lots of yeast and they taste yeasty. But they also do not give enough time for the bacteria to activate the lactic acid fermentation—this takes at least 48 hours to get going. This recipe uses yeast as a quick start, then ferments the dough in the refrigerator. You can use any type of whole wheat flour; I especially like white whole wheat for this recipe. For unbleached flour, I prefer Bob's Red Mill artisan bread flour.

MAKES 2 ROUND LOAVES (EACH LOAF IS 8 TO 10 SERVINGS)

PREP TIME: 5 MINUTES, PLUS 2 HOURS TO PROOF, 3 DAYS FOR FERMENTATION

BAKING TIME: 35 MINUTES

- 1 tablespoon active dry yeast
- 3½ cups white whole wheat flour
- 3 cups warm water (95°–105°F)
- 2½ teaspoons salt
- 3 cups unbleached all-purpose flour

1. In a large mixing bowl, mix the yeast and ½ cup of the warm water.
2. Add the whole wheat flour, the remaining 3 cups warm water, the salt, and the all-purpose flour, mixing while you add each to the bowl. Stir just enough to have all the flour absorbed, 2 to 3 minutes.
3. Cover the bowl with a thin fabric towel and let it sit out at room temperature for 2 hours.

4. Remove the towel, cover the bowl with plastic wrap, and place in the refrigerator for at least 3 days. The sourdough taste will get more pronounced the longer it sits (up to 2 weeks). My favorite time frame is 3 to 5 days.

5. When ready to bake, cut the dough in half to make two loaves. You can bake both one after the other or refrigerate the remaining loaf in an airtight container for up to 1 week. Place parchment paper on the counter, and using a little extra flour, work the dough into a ball for 1 to 2 minutes, without actually kneading.

6. Preheat the oven to 450°F and place a Dutch oven (without lid) on the middle rack of the oven. Let the bread rest for 30 minutes while the oven heats.

7. Slash an X in the top of the dough with a serrated knife, cutting about ½ inch deep. Set the dough in the hot Dutch oven and place the lid on top. Bake for 25 minutes.

8. Remove the lid, and bake an additional 12 to 15 minutes, until the top is golden brown. Remove bread from the pot and let it cool on a rack for at least 10 minutes before slicing.

GLUTEN-FREE OPTION: Use gluten-free flour
VEGAN OPTION: No modification needed
AIP OPTION: No option available

Greens, Alliums, and Cruciferous Veggies

If you have not had your quota for greens, alliums, and cruciferous vegetables for the day, here is a fast and tasty dish that will help you check off those boxes all at once! I like to have frozen spinach, broccoli florets, and some diced onions on hand so I can quickly assemble this side dish.

SERVES 4 **PREP TIME: 5 MINUTES** **TOTAL TIME: 20 MINUTES**

- 2 teaspoons salt
- 1 (12-ounce) bag frozen broccoli florets
- 1 (12-ounce) bag frozen chopped spinach
- 1 (10- or 12-ounce) bag frozen diced white onion
- 1 teaspoon extra-virgin olive oil
- Salt and freshly ground black pepper

1. Place 1 quart water in a large saucepan and fit with a steamer basket. Adjust the water level so that it is just below the steamer.
2. Add the salt to the water and bring to a simmer over medium-high heat, then reduce the heat to low.
3. Add the broccoli, spinach, and onion, and steam for roughly 10 minutes, or until the veggies are warmed through. Stir occasionally and add water, if needed.
4. Turn off the heat, carefully remove the steamer basket, and pour all the vegetables into a serving dish. Drizzle with the olive oil and season with salt and pepper.

GLUTEN-FREE OPTION: No modification needed
VEGAN OPTION: No modification needed
AIP OPTION: No modification needed

Roasted Garlic

We make this side dish a few times when my cousin's garlic is harvested in August or anytime fresh garlic at the store looks particularly fetching. This is also great if you feel a cold coming on. The cooking time will vary based on the size and age of your garlic bulbs. Here, the instruction is to cook until soft, but you can cook even longer for a caramelized flavor. This dish works well on a tray of raw vegetables for dipping, plus some cooked chicken or some homemade bread or polenta.

MAKES 4 SERVINGS **PREP TIME: 5 MINUTES** **TOTAL TIME: 50 TO 80 MINUTES**

- 6 to 8 heads of garlic

1. Preheat the oven to 350°F.
2. Cut off the top of the garlic heads, creating a ½-inch opening onto the cloves.
3. Wrap each garlic head in aluminum foil. Place on a baking sheet in the oven and bake for 45 to 75 minutes, until the garlic has a soft, paste-like consistency.
4. Let the garlic heads cool briefly, then remove the foil, and let sit for 5 minutes.
5. Squeeze the roasted garlic cloves into small serving bowls and serve with fresh sourdough bread or as an accompaniment to any vegetable dish.

GLUTEN-FREE OPTION: No modification needed
VEGAN OPTION: No modification needed
AIP OPTION: No option available

Thyroid Friendly Pesto

Basil comes in many varieties, including holy basil (*Ocimum tenuiflorum*) and culinary basil (*Ocimum basilicum*). Both types of basil are known to have antioxidant and immune-regulating properties, but the typical pesto has more cheese and oil than basil. This version is lighter, with a cleaner and more concentrated flavor. Aquafaba is the cooking or canning liquid for beans. With no flavor of its own, it is a perfect texturizer and source of resistant starch. If you have some home-cooked light-colored beans, just use of that liquid; otherwise, open a can of chickpeas and pour off ½ cup of the liquid (refrigerate the beans for later use). I love to serve pesto immediately after blending it. The colors and flavors start to darken or fade almost immediately. Serve this pesto over whole-grain pasta or zucchini noodles, along with a protein like diced chicken breast or sautéed crumbled tempeh.

MAKES ABOUT 1 CUP **PREP TIME: 10 MINUTES** **TOTAL TIME: 10 MINUTES**

- 4 ounces fresh basil leaves, stems removed
- 2 garlic cloves
- ½ cup liquid from beans
- Pinch of cayenne pepper
- 1 tablespoon fresh lemon juice, or more to taste
- Salt

1. Place the basil, garlic, bean liquid, cayenne, and 1 tablespoon lemon juice in a food processor or blender. Blend until smooth and bright green.
2. Add salt and, if desired, additional lemon juice. Serve immediately.

GLUTEN-FREE OPTION: No modification needed
VEGAN OPTION: No modification needed
AIP OPTION: Use water or bone broth instead of bean liquid and omit the cayenne

Pico de Gallo

This is a flavorful way to add zest to your veggies, protein, or carbs.

MAKES 1 CUP **PREP TIME: 5 MINUTES** **TOTAL TIME: 20 MINUTES**

- 4 ripe Roma (plum) tomatoes, finely chopped
- 1 medium onion, finely chopped
- 1 bunch fresh cilantro, finely chopped
- Juice of 1 lime
- 1 small jalapeño pepper, seeded and finely diced (optional)
- ½ teaspoon salt

1. In a medium bowl, combine the tomatoes, onion, and cilantro. Add the lime juice and jalapeño, if using. Add salt and mix thoroughly.
2. Let sit for at least 15 minutes so the flavors can meld.

SERVING SUGGESTION: Use as a fat-free salad dressing or spoon onto your fish or chicken entrée; you can also use to top off your beans

GLUTEN-FREE OPTION: No modification needed

VEGAN OPTION: No modification needed

AIP OPTION: No option available

DESSERTS

I don't normally serve dessert at home because we always have fruit on hand. If we're still a little hungry after eating, we'll grab a piece of fruit. Here are a few favorites for special occasions when you feel like having something extra.

Norwegian Amaranth Pudding

Okay, so my grandparents used white rice and cow's milk when they made this. They used to joke that all Norwegian food had to be white. Since I'm a fan of whole grains and amaranth makes such a great pudding, I altered the recipe to make this dish even more delicious.

SERVES 4 TO 6 **PREP TIME: 5 MINUTES** **TOTAL TIME: 55 MINUTES, PLUS 4 MORE HOURS TO CHILL**

- ½ cup amaranth grains
- 2 cups unflavored non-dairy milk (such as unsweetened flax milk)
- ½ teaspoon salt
- ½ teaspoon ground cardamom
- 1 teaspoon vanilla extract
- ⅓ cup dried red currants or raisins

1. In a large saucepan over high heat, bring 1½ cups water to a boil and add the amaranth. Cover, reduce the heat to medium low, and simmer for 30 minutes, stirring occasionally.

2. Add the non-dairy milk, salt, cardamom, vanilla, and currants, if using. Cover and simmer for 20 minutes more, stirring occasionally.

3. Chill for 4 or more hours before serving.

GLUTEN-FREE OPTION: No modification needed
VEGAN OPTION: No modification needed
AIP OPTION: No option available

Pistachio Chia Pudding

Did you enjoy pistachio ice cream before your dietary enlightenment? If so, here is a great substitute you can feel good about.

SERVES 4   **PREP TIME: 3 MINUTES**   **TOTAL TIME: 5 MINUTES**

- 1 cup unflavored non-dairy milk (such as unsweetened flax milk)
- 3 tablespoons chia seeds
- Sweetener, as desired (stevia or lo han)
- 1 teaspoon vanilla extract
- ¼ cup chopped pistachios, plus 2 tablespoons chopped for garnish
- 2 Medjool dates, pitted

1. In a blender, combine the non-dairy milk, chia seeds, sweetener, vanilla, ¼ cup pistachios, and dates. Blend for 1 to 2 minutes, or until smooth.
2. Pour into a bowl and refrigerate at least 1 hour.
3. Garnish with the chopped pistachios.

SERVING SUGGESTION: Because this is high in healthy fats, if weight control is an issue for you, skip the fats in your meal you are pairing this with

GLUTEN-FREE OPTION: No modification needed

VEGAN OPTION: No modification needed

AIP OPTION: No option available

Apple and Brazil Nut Cobbler

Here is another way to get your Brazil nuts. If you have already had yours for the day, you could use all pecans.

SERVES 5   PREP TIME: 30 MINUTES   TOTAL TIME: 1 HOUR, 40 MINUTES

- Avocado oil in a mister or nonstick cooking spray
- ¼ cup white whole wheat flour
- 2 tablespoon non-dairy spread (Smart Balance or Earth Balance brands)
- ½ cup old-fashioned rolled oats
- 4 Brazil nuts, chopped
- 2 tablespoons chopped pecans
- ⅓ cup allulose powder or other sweetener of choice
- ½ teaspoon salt
- 2½ pounds mildly sweet apples (McIntosh, Gala, Braeburn), cored and thinly sliced
- 1 tablespoon lemon juice

1. Preheat the oven to 350°F. Mist a 4 by 8-inch baking pan with the avocado oil.
2. In a medium bowl, combine the flour, lemon juice, non-dairy spread, oats, nuts, allulose powder, and salt.
3. Arrange the apple slices in the bottom of the baking pan. Sprinkle lemon juice over apple slices, then spread the cobbler mixture on top. Bake for 60 minutes, until the fruit is tender and the top is lightly browned.
4. Let cool for 15 minutes, then serve.

SERVING SUGGESTION: Because this is mostly carbs, have half your carb serving with whichever meal you eat this with

GLUTEN-FREE OPTION: Use gluten-free flour

VEGAN OPTION: No modification needed

AIP OPTION: Substitute ¾ cup almond flour for the whole wheat flour and rolled oats; substitute coconut oil for the spread

Chapter Nine

FAQ

Here they are: the thyroid questions I hear the most. I am happy to present them here as a chance to review them with you. In most cases, the answers come down to two things: fad diets are overblown, and food fears are unfounded.

Let's dive in. If I miss one of your questions, check out the sources, as I may have answered it elsewhere; if not, I'd love to help! I've included ways to get in touch with me at the end of this chapter.

WHAT IF NOTHING SEEMS TO BE WORKING?

The most common reason for this is that there was more iodine getting into your system than you expected. There are two ways to examine this, and they are not exclusive.

The first is to take a close look at all the possible sources of iodine in your life. It can be tempting to think that the occasional flavored coffee couldn't have that much iodine, or that there is just a little iodine in this multivitamin, but it is your favorite and you've taken it forever, so how could it be a problem? Be thorough. Be merciless. Give no quarter.

The other step is to check and see. You can test yourself and see how much iodine you've been exposed to. The results will show an average for the last three weeks. Taking a collection for the urinary iodine test is easy; it only requires a random urine collection. It does not require a sterile sample, and you don't have to fast beforehand. Some labs can run this test via a dried spot test, which means a collection can be made at home and mailed in. To find out how to run it, visit www.thyroidresetdiet.com/resources.

WHAT IF MY THYROID IS IMPROVING BUT I DON'T FEEL BETTER?

Over 84 percent of people with thyroid disease have another condition that contributes to their symptoms. It will take help from a doctor to get a proper diagnosis and treatment. To get started, here is a quick table that will give you get a sense of what else could be affecting you, based on your symptoms.

Note: Each of these conditions affects more than 5 percent of people with thyroid disease. They are all commonly underdiagnosed.

SYMPTOMS	POSSIBLE HIDDEN CAUSE	SCREENING TESTS
Fatigue	Anemia, heart disease, kidney disease	Routine blood tests—chemistry panel, iron panels
Insomnia	Sleep apnea	Home sleep apnea screen
Weight-loss resistance	Fatty liver, diabetes	Height-to-waist ratio, routine fasting blood tests, morning fasting glucose, A1C
Gas and bloating	Parathyroid disease, IBS, IBD	Routine blood tests—calcium levels, food intolerance test, stool culture
Hair loss	Anemia, PCOS	Iron panels, hormone tests, ovarian ultrasound
Pain	Arthritis, fibromyalgia	Physical exam, X-ray
Depression/anxiety	Adrenal, anemia, celiac obesity	Depression and anxiety symptom survey, cortisol slope test, iron panels, celiac screen

SHOULD I TRY TO LOWER MY ANTIBODIES?

People trying to correct thyroid disease talk about their goals in different ways. Some talk about going into remission, some talk about being cured, and others just talk about wanting to feel better.

Many people with thyroid disease focus on the goal of going into remission. Usually, this means that their thyroid antibodies have become no longer measurable. The assumption is that if the antibodies are not measurable, the disease is gone and they will finally feel better. The idea does make intuitive sense.

Many who have "gone into remission" still require thyroid medications and still have certain ongoing symptoms with which they struggle. Too many people have been led to think that having their thyroid antibodies go negative is the Holy Grail, the most important pursuit. Yet research shows that thyroid antibodies can go up and down in ways that do not seem to be significant. The ongoing levels of thyroid antibodies do not predict whether your thyroid will work by itself again, nor do they predict other things like risks for nodular growth or thyroid cancer.

Once a thyroid patient's antibody status is known, it is debatable as to whether there is any value in retesting it in the future.[1] Many with thyroid disease never even have medical antibodies to begin with, and if that same person retests his or her antibodies on the same day, the results will always vary.

There is also the fact that thyroid antibodies are not the cause of thyroid damage.[2] Many people with thyroid disease often find this surprising to hear. How can this be true if thyroid antibodies are part of the diagnosis of thyroid disease? I think a good analogy is that of smoke and fire. If someone's house is on fire, the first visible evidence is billowing smoke. Eliminating the smoke isn't going to quench the flames. This is exactly our current understanding of thyroid antibodies and thyroid glandular damage.

In another unexpected wrinkle, those who have positive thyroid peroxidase antibodies have lower risks for many cancers, including breast cancer, than those who do not.[3] Those with subclinical hypothyroidism and positive thyroid antibodies have no higher risk for developing overt hypothyroidism than similar patients do with negative thyroid antibodies.

I would encourage you to focus your energies on identifying any symptoms and have a goal of feeling as well as you did before the thyroid disease, if not better. For many people, thyroid function can improve, and they may not need to be on medication over the long term.

Your antibodies may go lower, they may fluctuate, or they may not change. Thankfully in most cases, the antibodies do not predict your likelihood of feeling better or having your thyroid work well again.

DOES HIGH-DOSE IODINE PREVENT BREAST CANCER?

The short answer is no. It is safer to be low iodine than high iodine. The consensus of the evidence suggests that having excessive iodine raises the risk of breast cancer. Some researchers have even suggested that urinary iodine levels could be used as a screen for determining who is at risk for breast cancer.[4]

A 2003 study asked whether there could be some link between iodine intake and breast cancer risk. One link that emerged surprised many people. It turns out that having positive thyroid antibodies seems to be protective against breast cancer.[5] The rates of breast cancer among Japanese women are low and their dietary intake of sea vegetables is high, yet their rate of thyroid disease is elevated.

One of the more recent papers to address this issue found that those with the lowest iodine levels had one-third the breast cancer risk as those with normal or higher iodine levels.[6] There is no danger of higher breast cancer risk with a low-iodine diet. If anything, it appears to be protective.

SHOULD I GO GLUTEN-FREE?

If you have celiac disease or a wheat allergy, you must go gluten-free. If you are gluten-free for other reasons and you wish to stay that way,

I have no desire to talk you out of it. Studies are suggesting that those who are gluten-free have worse health outcomes than those who are not, as in cardiovascular death and obesity.[7] Those concerns also seem to apply to those with celiac disease as likely healthier if they eat gluten-free whole grains.[8] However, it seems that the harm comes more from avoiding whole grains entirely than from avoiding gluten. You can likely include gluten-free whole grains and still be healthy.

Some writers have implicated gluten as causing thyroid disease, since many people with celiac disease also have thyroid disease. It is thought that somehow reactions to gluten caused thyroid disease in ways that may be relevant for those without celiac. As the studies evolved, we learned that celiac does not cause thyroid disease; rather, some underlying susceptibility to autoimmunity gives rise to both. We know this because we have seen that whether those newly diagnosed go gluten-free or not, their rates of developing thyroid disease are the same.[9] We also know that for those who have celiac disease and thyroid disease, going gluten-free is important, but it does not improve thyroid function.[10]

Yet many people with thyroid disease report that going gluten-free has helped improve their thyroid function. This observation could be more than a misattribution. People on typical diets get most of their gluten from commercially baked goods—breads, bagels, rolls, biscuits, muffins, cakes, and cookies.

If you have thyroid disease, I do encourage screening for celiac disease with blood tests. The Thyroid Reset Diet does avoid processed sources of gluten and is easy to follow for those who are gluten-free.

SHOULD I AVOID GOITROGENS?

Foods contain a variety of compounds that, in isolation, could slow the activity of the thyroid gland. Many thyroid diets focus efforts on identifying and avoiding many of the known goitrogens found in soy or cruciferous vegetables.

The three possibly goitrogenic compounds found in food include glucosinolates from cruciferous vegetables; polyphenols from tea, chocolate, apples, and others, and a subtype of polyphenols called isoflavones from soy, flax, and many other foods; and perchlorate from many foods and water supplies. All these have been thoroughly studied in humans, and except for perchlorates from water supplies, none is relevant in the amounts found in the human diet.

Before 1991, when there were more countries at iodine level 1 (see Chapter Four), high amounts of dietary goitrogens could be relevant for people who lived in those areas. At present, in the modern world, they simply are not relevant. Furthermore, the same compounds that are goitrogenic are generally health-promoting for other reasons.

GLUCOSINOLATES

These are found in varying amounts in cruciferous vegetables, such as:

- Arugula
- Bok choy
- Broccoli
- Broccoli rabe
- Brussels sprouts
- Cabbage
- Cauliflower
- Chinese cabbage
- Collard greens
- Daikon
- Kale
- Mustard
- Radish
- Rutabaga
- Turnips
- Watercress

A placebo-controlled double-blind study with volunteers was done to see if high-dose glucosinolates extracted from broccoli sprouts could cause a measurable change in thyroid function. The volunteers did a five-day diet with minimal amounts of cruciferous vegetables, followed by doses of broccoli sprout extract every eight hours for 21 doses. Each dose contained either 25 or 100 units of sulforaphane; the lower amount is equivalent to over 4 pounds of broccoli. No detrimental effects were noted on any thyroid markers or liver function on either dose. TSH scores improved in those in the group given sulforaphane.[11]

POLYPHENOLS

Despite being categorized as goitrogenic, dietary polyphenols have been shown to correlate with lower rates of autoimmune thyroid disease.

ISOFLAVONES

These are a subgroup of polyphenols that contain estrogen regulating compounds. They are found in many foods including soy, flax, chickpeas, pistachios, peanuts, red clover, chocolate, and fava beans.[12]

A recent comprehensive analysis of all known research on soy and thyroid disease concluded that soy isoflavones have no relevant effects on thyroid function.[13]

PERCHLORATE

Perchlorate is a naturally occurring compound found in many dietary sources and from groundwater.

Many of the U.S. water supplies are contaminated with perchlorate. In an analysis of 3,262 homes, 83 percent were found to have measurable perchlorate. It is thought to be present in twenty-six states, two territories, and in water systems that supply water to 11 million people. At present, the EPA does not regulate perchlorate in drinking water.[14]

Among the areas with the highest perchlorate levels are those supplied water from the Colorado River—much of the southwestern United States, including Arizona and California. In these regions, urinary perchlorate levels are often two times higher than national averages.[15]

Perchlorate has a known inhibitory effect on thyroid function. In the past, it was used as a treatment for hyperthyroidism before current treatments with fewer side effects were available.[16] Studies have shown that low-level perchlorate exposure can increase rates of thyroid disease in populations, but this effect has been refuted by some studies. The amount of perchlorate found in foods does not seem to be relevant, but the amount found in water can be in areas in which it is highest.

As a goitrogen, perchlorate is worth being aware of as a reason to avoid unpurified water for those who have or are concerned about thyroid disease. If you are drinking purified water, perchlorate is not a concern.

SHOULD I GO KETOGENIC?

If extreme diets slow thyroid hormone production, are ketogenic diets any different? Is there some way that high amounts of ketones compensate for the negative effects of low-carbohydrate or low-protein diets on thyroid function?

It is important to first differentiate the effects of total food intake from the effects of avoiding certain food categories. When total food intake is lowered, it is common to see a short-term reduction in markers of inflammation, such as thyroid antibodies going down temporarily when they are already present. Based on the known mechanisms of insulin on thyroid production, one would expect ketogenic diets to have deleterious effects on the thyroid since they often lower insulin well below the low end of healthy ranges.

The only published information we have on ketogenic diets and thyroid function do bear this out. There are no interventional trials but there are data from children who were put on ketogenic diets for epilepsy and subsequently monitored for changes in thyroid function.

Thyroid disease among children is rare and epileptic children are not more prone to thyroid disease than children without epilepsy. Clinicians guiding children through ketogenic diets were noticing an unusually high rate of thyroid disease and decided to track it to see if it was a trend. Two published studies are looking at this association. Both showed that ketogenic diets caused negative changes to thyroid function.

The rate of hypothyroidism among preadolescent children is roughly 1 in 1,250, or about 0.08 percent.[17] As part of this study, one in six of the children became hypothyroid and required thyroid replacement therapy. Due to these findings, the researchers concluded that the diet itself caused thyroid malfunction. Ultimately, they suggested that thyroid function should be monitored regularly in those with epilepsy who were on the ketogenic diet.[18]

Adults may have different responses from children, but given that they are more prone to thyroid disease, it would not be rational to expect them to fare better. It is important to note that ketogenic diets currently have a place for children with epilepsy that does not respond to medications. My inclusion of these studies should not discourage parents from considering the approach when advised by a neurologist and supervised registered dietician.

WHAT IF I GET TOO LITTLE IODINE?

What if you follow the Thyroid Reset Diet and end up with health problems stemming from iodine deficiency? How can you be sure you will not be getting too little iodine?

One of the unique things about iodine as a nutrient is that it plays a singular role in the body and that role is all about thyroid function. Many believe that it is the single most researched nutrient. With everything we know about it, there are no other ways it is known to be relevant.

Once your iodine levels are healthy for your thyroid, they are healthy for the rest of you. Every part of your body depends on the right number of thyroid hormones to work well, but for every part besides your thyroid, iodine deficiency has no direct effects. Some have claimed that iodine is directly essential for breast health. For more on iodine and breast health, please see the earlier question "Does High-Dose Iodine Prevent Breast Cancer?"

Numerous animal and human studies have looked at the question of whether iodine intake is significant to those with normal thyroid function. The consensus is that it is not.

Iodine requirements are different for children and for pregnant or nursing women. In these cases, please consult with your personal physician for guidance.

CAN I USE THE THYROID RESET DIET AS A LOW-IODINE DIET?

Suppose you have been recommended to follow a low-iodine diet to prepare for an iodine uptake scan or radioiodine ablation. Does the Thyroid Reset Diet count as a low-iodine diet?

Yes, the Reset phase of the Thyroid Reset Diet and its recipes can safely be used to follow low-iodine diet recommendations in preparation for iodine uptake scan studies or radioactive iodine ablation treatments. Stick with Green Light foods and you will do fine. Be sure to follow the guidelines for avoiding all vitamins containing iodine including multivitamins and those for using iodine-free salt.

HOW IS THE THYROID RESET DIET DIFFERENT FROM A LOW-IODINE DIET?

The low-iodine diet intentionally lowers the daily iodine intake to under 40 mcg in total. This makes the 2 mcg of radioactive iodine 5 percent of the total daily intake, or twelve times more concentrated.

The typical duration of the low-iodine diet is two weeks before a procedure. Evidence shows that a single week is usually adequate, but most people require the first week to get consistent with the new diet. Because the diet is for a brief period, and because it intends to drastically reduce iodine, it cuts out many food categories.

These include:

- Iodized salt or any salt not defined as non-iodized
- Sea salt
- Artificially colored foods, due to FD&C Red Dye #3 being a high source of iodine
- All dairy products
- All products containing egg yolks
- All baked goods unless homemade with non-iodized salt and no iodine-based dough conditioners
- All soy products

- Molasses and brown sugar
- Foods with carrageenan, agar-agar, algin, or alginates
- Any sea vegetables
- Any supplements with iodine
- Any medications with iodine
- In some versions, animal protein is limited to 1 small serving per day. In other versions, it is not.[19]

The low-iodine diet can make it hard to get adequate amounts of micronutrients such as those found in dairy foods like calcium, riboflavin, and vitamins A and D; and those in seafood like the omega 3 fats EPA and DHA. However, due to the brief duration, this is less of a concern.

DO PARASITES LIKE *BLASTOCYSTIS HOMINIS* CAUSE THYROID DISEASE?

Many have wondered if certain parasites can cause thyroid disease. In addition to *B. hominis*, others proposed have included *Entamoeba histolytica*, *Giardia lamblia*, cryptosporidium, hookworm, and pinworm.

I focus this discussion on *B. hominis* since most literature is about it, but the conclusions fit the others as well. If you do have symptoms of parasitic infection, such as new-onset gas, bloating, irregular stools, bloody diarrhea, do screen for parasites as part of the diagnostic process if these symptoms persist. Work with your doctor to treat any foreign organisms that show up on your stool studies.

What about those who have no digestive symptoms, or perhaps they do but they have come and gone for some time? Should these people screen for parasites because they have thyroid disease? Furthermore, if you are in this situation and you did have parasites show up on a nontraditional test, should you take herbs or medications to eradicate it?

In these situations, no evidence suggests that such treatment would help your thyroid. It is important to note that most parasitic treatments do cause side effects, and many can cause harm.

SHOULD I AVOID SOY?

Please do avoid soy if you have a soy allergy or if you are avoiding soy to adhere to soy-free diet guidelines, such as those in AIP diets.

Otherwise, soy is safe for your thyroid. Many do claim that soy is harmful to thyroid function; some say it is less so if it is fermented. The largest study to date was done in 2019 and it reviewed all the studies to date on soy and thyroid function. They included all studies that looked at the effects of soy or soy constituents like genistein or daidzein and their impact on thyroid disease or any blood markers of thyroid function in adult humans.

They concluded that "soy supplementation has no effect on the thyroid hormones."[20] I've looked at much of this literature. The concerns stemmed from the first infant formulas made with soy protein. These had been in use since 1909 for babies who had dairy allergies and did not have access to breast milk.

In the late 1950s, researchers identified an increased rate of goiter among infants on soy formulas. It was found that soy protein has a stronger effect on binding to iodine than milk protein does. Since these infants were consuming food from no other sources, they became iodine deficient even though they were supplemented with iodine.

When the problem was identified in 1959, the amount of iodine in the formula was simply adjusted to compensate for the binding. Soy flour was also replaced with soy protein isolate. The binding issue can happen anytime minerals and proteins are mixed. Dairy formulas bind iron more strongly than do soy formulas, therefore more iron is needed to compensate.

Some claim that the increased goiter rate was related to constituents in soy, such as isoflavones or trypsin inhibitors. Yet even though these elements are still in place, soy formulas no longer cause higher rates of goiter.[21]

I think the soy topic is important because choosing to avoid it is not a neutral choice. The evidence is solid that including soy in the diet can benefit many issues important to the demographics prone to thyroid disease: women in their premenopausal and post-menopausal years. Some are surprised to learn that soy can decrease the severity of menopausal symptoms,[22] lower the risk of brain aging and heart disease,[23] lower the risk of osteoporosis,[24] lower the risk of breast cancer, and lower the risk of recurrence in those who have had breast cancer.[25]

SHOULD I SUPPLEMENT WITH VITAMIN D?

Vitamin D is an essential nutrient we can get from our diets, the sun, or from supplements.

The most significant dietary source is dairy foods that are fortified with vitamin D. Since the Thyroid Reset Diet is lower in dairy foods, dietary sources of vitamin D are generally lacking. There is no doubt that those who are diligent about sun exposure can achieve adequate vitamin D blood levels from it alone.

For sunlight to work for vitamin D, you need to be out in prime hours, 10 a.m. to 2 p.m., or when your shadow is shorter than you. The duration can be tricky. It may range from 10 to 90 minutes based on latitude, as well as pigmentation, amount of skin exposure, and amount of body fat. Body fat traps vitamin D and leaves less available for circulation. Those with more body fat need more vitamin D for the same serum levels.

Many find that they are often not exposed to the sun enough for skin production of vitamin D to bring them to the best levels. For most, vitamin D supplementation is helpful. The safest blood levels for overall health appear to be in a narrow part of the lower end of the range, or roughly 30 to 50 ng/ml.[26]

A good starting dose is 1,000 IU daily. Check vitamin D levels after six months to get back into range and annually thereafter. You may see recommendations claiming that those with autoimmune disease should have vitamin D levels as high as 50 to 120 ng/ml. I do not agree because levels this high are related to a higher risk of heart disease and mortality and it is not clear that higher levels justify the risk.[27,28]

In Closing

Thank you for picking up this book. I believe books have the power to change our lives more than any other medium.

This book will best help your thyroid journey when used along with its companion software: The Personalized Thyroid Plan. This is an interactive training program that can give you specific guidance based on your needs for each step of the journey. I've never seen anything like it before and I'm excited to share it. You can find it on the resources page www.thyroidresetdiet.com/resources.

If you are a practitioner, much of what I wanted to put in here is more for you. Visit the resources page to find out about practitioner training options.

You can do so much better in the world when your body and mind don't hold you back. Hold on to your dream of vibrant and joyous health. Be a role model for others and share with them what you learn.

Let's stay connected. If you do have more questions, you can ask them in person and join me for "Office Hours Live" almost every Monday at 4 p.m. AZ time. (We don't follow daylight saving time.) I'm on both Facebook and Instagram @dralanchristianson.

To your best health,

Dr. C

Shopping Lists

Here are the shopping lists for each week. At first you will want to stock up on the staples, but after that you'll mostly just need to get perishables like produce and protein. Some items do not come in small enough sizes to exactly fit so you may have some items left over after each week.

If you'd like to print a copy and bring it with you, you can find a printer friendly version on the resources page www.thyroidresetdiet.com/resources.

THYROID RESET KITCHEN STAPLES

These pantry items are things you don't have to buy every week. Keep any or all of them in your pantry so you can create most meals. You don't need them all. And you most likely already have many in your kitchen.

If you start to make a meal and find you don't have a particular ingredient, you can often replace it with something else from the list or leave it out entirely. It truly is up to you.

PANTRY PROTEINS

- Protein powder: pea, hemp (assayed for low-iodine content), vanilla, or unflavored
- Canned chicken breast
- Dried lentils, red, orange

PANTRY FATS

- Grapeseed oil, extra-virgin olive oil, avocado oil, toasted sesame oil
- Sunflower seeds, sesame seeds, pumpkin seeds, chia seeds
- Brazil nuts, almonds, cashews (all unsalted)
- Organic nut butters

PANTRY CARBS

- Rice: brown, wild, long-grain white; quinoa, millet, freekeh
- Grains: old-fashioned rolled oats; buckwheat groats
- Beans (unsalted): pinto, navy, black, cannellini, chickpeas; bean soup mix
- Pasta: whole-grain penne, buckwheat soba and udon noodles
- Flour: buckwheat, whole wheat, bread, all-purpose; baking powder

EXTRACTS, SPICES, CONDIMENTS

- Cocoa powder, natural unsweetened or Dutch-process; carob (toasted or plain)
- Mint extract, orange extract, vanilla extract, and so on
- Mustard, stone-ground, Dijon; tamari; capers; canned green chiles; olives; anchovies
- Non-iodized salt; black and white pepper; dried herbs: basil, oregano, herbes de Provence, Italian seasoning blend, bouquet garni; spices: ground cardamom, cloves, curry, cumin, smoked and regular paprika; nutmeg, allspice, cayenne pepper, chili powder, red pepper flakes, garam

masala, pumpkin pie spice, cinnamon, garlic powder, onion powder, turmeric, ginger, red curry paste
- Canned artichoke hearts (in water); canned unsalted tomatoes, crushed, diced; unsalted tomato paste; pumpkin puree
- Vinegars: red wine, white wine, ume plum, sherry, rice, balsamic
- Unsalted broth: chicken, beef, vegetable; powdered bouillon
- Miscellaneous: miso paste, nutritional yeast, arrowroot powder, sorghum grain, spirulina powder
- Sweeteners: honey, stevia, lo han

WEEK 1

REFRIGERATED ITEMS

1 (32-ounce) container unflavored non-dairy milk
1 (24-ounce) container non-dairy yogurt
1 dozen large eggs
1 (16-ounce) container liquid egg whites
1 (8-ounce) package grated parmesan cheese
1 block tempeh

MEAT AND SEAFOOD

1 (12.5-ounce) can canned chicken breast
1 (3- to 4-pound) roasting chicken
2 pounds skinless boneless chicken breasts
1 pound lean ground turkey
1 pound medium shrimp, shelled
2 pounds squid (calamari)

PRODUCE

5 medium red onions and 1 small red onion; 2 medium and 2 large yellow onions; 1 small white onion
2 heads garlic
1 shallot
1 bunch scallions
1 pound Yukon Gold potatoes
2 purple potatoes
2 sweet potatoes
2 medium carrots
1 bunch celery
2 fennel bulbs
3 bunches bok choy
1 head green cabbage
1 bunch fresh spinach
1 beefsteak tomato
7 Roma (plum) tomatoes
2 cucumbers
1 (8-ounce) package fresh button mushrooms
1 green bell pepper
2 ears corn
1 (16-ounce) package fresh green beans
1 medium zucchini
1 medium avocado
3 heads romaine lettuce
3 heads butter lettuce
1 loose head red-leaf lettuce
1 bunch arugula
1 bunch fresh parsley
1 bunch fresh chives
1 bunch fresh cilantro
1 bunch fresh basil
1 bunch fresh thyme
1 bunch fresh tarragon

FRUITS

1 pound frozen cherries
1 pint fresh blueberries
3 bananas
1 (8+-ounce) package seedless green grapes
1 lemon
2 limes
6 Medjool dates

OTHER

1 (8-ounce) package raw cashews

WEEK 2

REFRIGERATED ITEMS

1 (32-ounce) container unflavored non-dairy milk
1 dozen large eggs
1 (16-ounce) container liquid egg whites
1 block extra-firm tofu

MEAT AND SEAFOOD

1 (12.5-ounce) can chicken breast
1 pound lean ground turkey
2 pounds skinless boneless chicken breasts
1 pound extra-lean beef stew meat
1½ pounds lean ground beef (93 percent)
1 pound medium shrimp, shelled

PRODUCE

5 medium and 1 small red onions; 7 medium white onions
1 shallot
1 bunch scallions
4 heads garlic
3½ pounds Yukon Gold potatoes
6 russet potatoes
6 medium carrots
1 (8-ounce) package baby carrots
1 bunch celery
2 cucumbers
1 (8-ounce) package fresh button mushrooms
1 head cauliflower
1 fennel bulb
9 Roma (plum) tomatoes
1 pint cherry tomatoes
2 beefsteak tomatoes
1 (16-ounce) package fresh green beans
1 red bell pepper
2 jalapeño peppers
1 serrano chile
1 pound tomatillos
1 knob fresh ginger
1 (8-ounce) package fresh spinach
1 (8-ounce) package fresh kale
1 (8-ounce) package snow peas
3 medium avocados
5 heads butter lettuce
1 head romaine lettuce
1 loose head red-leaf lettuce
1 bunch fresh basil
1 bunch fresh thyme
1 bunch fresh parsley
1 bunch fresh oregano
4 bunches fresh cilantro

FRUITS

2 peaches
1 banana
1 pear
1 Granny Smith apple
1 (8+-ounce) package seedless green grapes
1 orange
5 limes
1 lemon
4 Medjool dates

OTHER

1 (1-ounce) package whole almonds

WEEK 3

REFRIGERATED ITEMS

1 (24-ounce) container unflavored non-dairy yogurt
1 (32-ounce) container unflavored non-dairy milk
1 dozen large eggs
1 (16-ounce) container liquid egg whites
1 (16-ounce container) extra-firm tofu
1 (8-ounce) container miso paste
1 (8-ounce) package grated parmesan cheese

MEAT AND SEAFOOD

1 (12.5-ounce) can chicken breast
2 pounds skinless boneless chicken breasts
2 pounds lean ground beef (93%)
1 pound lean ground turkey
1 pound river trout fillets (fresh or frozen)
1 pound catfish fillets

PRODUCE

1 medium yellow onion; 4 medium red onions; 1 medium sweet onion; 1 small white onion
2 bunches green bulbing onions
3 heads garlic
1 shallot
1 pound Yukon Gold potatoes
2 sweet potatoes
1 head green cabbage
3 baby bok choy
1 fennel bulb
1 bunch celery
1 bunch spinach leaves
1 cucumber
1 (8-ounce) package fresh shiitake mushrooms
1 (8-ounce) package fresh button mushrooms
1 (8-ounce) package sugar snap peas
1 (16-ounce) package French-cut green beans
1 (16-ounce) package green beans
1 (8-ounce) package snow peas
2 red bell peppers
1 beefsteak tomato
2 Roma (plum) tomatoes
1 pint cherry tomatoes
5 heads butter lettuce
3 heads romaine lettuce
1 bunch arugula
1 knob fresh ginger
1 kabocha winter squash (2 to 3 pounds)
1 medium zucchini
1 bunch fresh parsley
1 bunch fresh thyme
2 bunches fresh basil
1 bunch fresh oregano
1 bunch fresh cilantro

FRUITS

1 pint fresh blueberries
1 pint fresh blackberries
3 navel oranges
1 Granny Smith apple
1 pear
2 lemons
1 lime
2 bananas

OTHER

1 (4-ounce) can of green chilis
1 (12-ounce) box whole-grain penne pasta
1 (10-ounce) can unsalted diced tomatoes

WEEK 4

REFRIGERATED ITEMS

1 (32-ounce) container unflavored non-dairy milk
1 (24-ounce) container unflavored non-dairy yogurt
1 dozen large eggs
1 (16-ounce) container liquid egg whites
1 (12-ounce) package tempeh

MEAT AND SEAFOOD

1 (12.5-ounce) can chicken breast
1 (3- to 4-pound) roasting chicken
2 pounds skinless boneless chicken breasts
1 pound lean ground turkey
1 pound halibut fillet
1 pound medium shrimp, shelled

PRODUCE

3 medium red onions; 1 large and 5 medium yellow onions
3 heads garlic
1 shallot
2 bunches scallions
1 bunch celery
3 medium carrots
10 to 11 Yukon Gold potatoes
4 purple potatoes
3 baby bok choy
1 head cauliflower
1 bunch broccoli
1 (8-ounce) package fresh button mushrooms
1 (8-ounce) package fresh shiitake mushrooms
1 knob fresh ginger
2 stalks fresh lemongrass
3 bunches fresh spinach
1 bunch fresh kale
1 (8-ounce) package sugar snap peas
2 pounds fresh green beans
1 beefsteak tomato
3 Roma (plum) tomatoes
4 heads butter lettuce
1 loose head red-leaf lettuce
1 bunch arugula
3 medium avocados
3 bunches fresh cilantro
1 bunch fresh tarragon
1 bunch fresh mint
1 bunch fresh basil
1 bunch fresh thyme
1 bunch fresh oregano
1 (10-ounce) package frozen peas
1 pint cherry tomatoes
2 red bell peppers

FRUIT

2 small to medium apples
4 bananas
1 orange
1 lemon
2 limes

Notes

INTRODUCTION

1. Yoon SJ, Choi SR, Kim DM, et al. The Effect of Iodine Restriction on Thyroid Function in Patients with Hypothyroidism Due to Hashimoto's Thyroiditis. *Yonsei Med J.* 2003;44(2):44–227.
2. Luo Y, Kawashima A, Ishido Y, et al. Iodine Excess as an Environmental Risk Factor for Autoimmune Thyroid Disease. *Int J Mol Sci.* 2014;15(7):12895–12912. doi:10.3390/ijms150712895
3. Iodine Global Network. Global Scorecard 2014: Number of Iodine Deficient Countries More Than Halved in Past Decade. IDD Newsletter.

CHAPTER ONE

1. American Thyroid Association. American Thyroid Association (ATA) Issues Statement on the Potential Risks of Excess Iodine Ingestion and Exposure. *Thyroid.* June 5, 2013.
2. Furszyfer J, Kurland LT, Woolner LB, Elveback LR, McConahey WM. Hashimoto's Thyroiditis in Olmsted County, Minnesota, 1935 through 1967. *Mayo Clin Proc.* 1970;45(8):586–596.

3. Duntas LH. The Catalytic Role of Iodine Excess in Loss of Homeostasis in Autoimmune Thyroiditis. *Curr Opin Endocrinol Diabetes Obes*. 2018;25(5):347–352. doi:10.1097/MED.0000000000000425

4. Peterson SJ, Cappola AR, Castro MR, et al. An Online Survey of Hypothyroid Patients Demonstrates Prominent Dissatisfaction. *Thyroid*. 2018;28(6):707–721. doi:10.1089/thy.2017.0681

5. Pehrsson PR, Patterson KY, Spungen JH, et al. Iodine in Food- and Dietary Supplement—Composition Databases. *Am J Clin Nutr*. 2016;104 (Suppl 3):868S–876S. doi:10.3945/ajcn.115.110064

6. Prevention of Iodine Deficiency; Prevention of Micronutrient Deficiencies. NCBI Bookshelf. https://www.ncbi.nlm.nih.gov/books/NBK230108/. Accessed May 14, 2020.

CHAPTER TWO

1. Ahad F, Ganie SA. Iodine, Iodine Metabolism and Iodine Deficiency Disorders Revisited. *Indian J Endocrinol Metab*. 2010;14(1):13–17.

2. Robbani I, Dhaar GM. *Foundations of Community Medicine*. Noida, Uttar Pradesh, India: Elsevier, 2008.

3. Heinrich TW, Grahm G. Hypothyroidism Presenting as Psychosis: Myxedema Madness Revisited. *Prim Care Companion J Clin Psychiatry*. 2003;5(6):260–266. doi:10.4088/pcc.v05n0603

CHAPTER THREE

1. Rhee CM, Bhan I, Alexander EK, Brunelli SM. Association between Iodinated Contrast Media Exposure and Incident Hyperthyroidism and Hypothyroidism. *Arch Intern Med*. 2012;172(2):153–159. doi:10.1001/archinternmed.2011.677

2. Leung AM, Braverman LE. Consequences of Excess Iodine. *Nat Rev*. 2014;10(3):136–142. doi:10.1038/nrendo.2013.251

3. Markou K, Georgopoulos N, Kyriazopoulou V, Vagenakis AG. Iodine-Induced Hypothyroidism. *Thyroid*. 2001;11(5):501–510. doi:10.1089/105072501300176462

4. Bagchi N, Brown TR, Urdanivia E, Sundick RS. Induction of Autoimmune Thyroiditis in Chickens by Dietary Iodine. *Sci (New York)*. 1985;230(4723):325–327. doi:10.1126/science.4048936

5. Champion BR, Rayner DC, Byfield PG, Page KR, Chan CT, Roitt IM. Critical Role of Iodination for T Cell Recognition of Thyroglobulin in Experimental Murine Thyroid Autoimmunity. *J Immunol*. 1987;139(11):3665–3670.

6. Many CM, Maniratunga S, Varis I, Dardenne M, Drexhage HA, Denef JF. Two-Step Development of Hashimoto-Like Thyroiditis in Genetically Autoimmune Prone Non-Obese Diabetic Mice: Effects of Iodine-Induced Cell Necrosis. *J Endocrinol*. 1995;147(2):311–320. doi:10.1677/joe.0.1470311

7. Braley-Mullen H, Sharp G, Medling B, Tang H. Spontaneous Autoimmune Thyroiditis in NOD.H–2h4 Mice. *J Autoimmun*. 1999;12(3):157–165. doi:10.1006/jaut.1999.0272

8. Luo Y, Kawashima A, Ishido Y, et al. Iodine Excess as an Environmental Risk Factor for Autoimmune Thyroid Disease. *Int J Mol Sci*. 2014;15(7):12895–12912.

9. Kawashima A, Tanigawa K, Akama T, Yoshihara A, Ishii N, Suzuki K. Innate Immune Activation and Thyroid Autoimmunity. *J Clin Endocrinol Metab*. 2011;96(12):3661–3671. doi:10.1210/jc.2011-1568

10. Kawashima A, Tanigawa K, Akama T, et al. Fragments of Genomic DNA Released by Injured Cells Activate Innate Immunity and Suppress Endocrine Function in the Thyroid. *Endocrinology*. 2011;152(4):1702–1712. doi:10.1210/en.2010-1132

11. Katagiri R, Yuan X, Kobayashi S, Sasaki S. Effect of Excess Iodine Intake on Thyroid Diseases in Different Populations: A Systematic Review and Meta-Analyses Including Observational Studies. *PLoS One*. 2017;12(3):e0173722. doi:10.1371/journal.pone.0173722

12. Hartstock CL. Iodized Salt in the Prevention of Goiter: Is It a Safe Measure for General Use? *JAMA*. 1926;86(18):1334–1338. doi:10.1001/jama.1926.02670440008005

13. Sun X, Shan Z, Teng W. Effects of Increased Iodine Intake on Thyroid Disorders. *Endocrinol Metab*. 2014;29:240–247. doi:10.3803/EnM.2014.29.3.240

14. Ghent WR, Eskin BA, Low DA, Hill LP. Iodine Replacement in Fibrocystic Disease of the Breast. *Can J Surg*. 1993;36(5):453–460.

15. Connelly KJ, Boston BA, Pearce EN, et al. Congenital hypothyroidism caused by excess prenatal maternal iodine ingestion. *J Pediatr*. 2012;161(4):760–762. doi:10.1016/j.jpeds.2012.05.057

16. Hoang TD, Mai VQ, Clyde PW, Shakir MK. Over-the-Counter-Drug-Induced Thyroid Disorders. *Endocr Pract*. 2013;19(2):268–274. doi:10.4158/EP12298.OR

17. Connelly KJ, Boston BA, Pearce EN, et al. Congenital Hypothyroidism Caused by Excess Prenatal Maternal Iodine Ingestion. *J Pediatr*. 2012;161(4):760–762. doi:10.1016/j.jpeds.2012.05.057

18. Sang Z, Wang PP, Yao Z, et al. Exploration of the Safe Upper Level of Iodine Intake in Euthyroid Chinese Adults: A Randomized Double-Blind Trial. *Am J Clin Nutr*. 2012;95(2):367–373. doi:10.3945/ajcn.111.028001

19. Kahaly G, Dienes HP, Beyer J, Hommel G. Randomized, Double Blind, Placebo-Controlled Trial of Low Dose Iodide in Endemic Goiter. *J Clin Endocrinol Metab*. 1997;82(12):4049–4053. doi:10.1210/jcem.82.12.4416

20. Kasagi K, Iwata M, Misaki T, Konishi J. Effect of Iodine Restriction on Thyroid Function in Patients with Primary Hypothyroidism. *Thyroid*. 2003;13(6):561–567. doi:10.1089/105072503322238827

CHAPTER FOUR

1. Iodine Global Network. Global Scorecard 2014: Number of Iodine Deficient Countries More Than Halved in Past Decade. IDD Newsletter.
2. Andersson M, Takkouche B, Egli I, Allen HE, de Benoist B. Current Global Iodine Status and Progress over the Last Decade towards the Elimination of Iodine Deficiency. *Bull World Health Organ.* 2005;83(7):518–525.
3. Hollowell JG, Haddow JE. The Prevalence of Iodine Deficiency in Women of Reproductive Age in the United States of America. *Public Health Nutr.* 2007;10(12A):1532–1539. doi:10.1017/S1368980007360862
4. Pearce EN, Pino S, He X, Bazrafshan HR, Lee SL, Braverman LE. Sources of Dietary Iodine: Bread, Cows' Milk, and Infant Formula in the Boston Area. *J Clin Endocrinol Metab.* 2004;89(7):3421–3424. doi:10.1210/jc.2003-032002
5. Lee KW, Shin D, Cho MS, Song WO. Food Group Intakes as Determinants of Iodine Status among U.S. Adult Population. *Nutrients.* 2016;8(6):325. doi:10.3390/nu8060325
6. Laurberg P, Pedersen KM, Hreidarsson A, Sigfusson N, Iversen E, Knudsen PR. Iodine Intake and the Pattern of Thyroid Disorders: A Comparative Epidemiological Study of Thyroid Abnormalities in the Elderly in Iceland and in Jutland, Denmark. *J Clin Endocrinol Metab.* 1998;83(3):765–769. doi:10.1210/jcem.83.3.4624
7. Schöne F, Spörl K, Leiterer M. Iodine in the Feed of Cows and in the Milk with a View to the Consumer's Iodine Supply. *J Trace Elem Med Biol.* 2017;39:202–209. doi:10.1016/j.jtemb.2016.10.004
8. BBC Radio 4—In Their Element, Series 2, Awesome Iodine. https://www.bbc.co.uk/programmes/b09plrg0. Accessed September 21, 2020.
9. Payling L, Juniper DT, Drake C. Effect of Milk Type and Processing on Iodine Concentration of Organic and Conventional Winter Milk at Retail: Implications for Nutrition. *Food Chem.* 2015;178. doi:10.1016/j.foodchem.2015.01.091
10. Stevenson MC, Drake C, Givens DI. Further Studies on the Iodine Concentration of Conventional, Organic and UHT Semi-Skimmed Milk at Retail in the UK. *Food Chem.* 2018;239:551–555. doi:10.1016/j.foodchem.2017.06.135
11. Pehrsson PR, Patterson KY, Spungen JH, et al. Iodine in Food and Dietary Supplement—Composition Databases. *Am J Clin Nutr.* 2016;104(Suppl 3):868S-76S. doi:10.3945/ajcn.115.110064
12. Nerhus I, Markhus MW, Nilsen BM, et al. Iodine Content of Six Fish Species, Norwegian Dairy Products, and Hen's Egg. *Food Nutr Res.* 2018;62. doi:10.29219/fnr.v62.1291
13. Hosomi R, Yoshida M, Fukunaga K. Seafood Consumption and Components for Health. *Glob J Health Sci.* 2012;4(3):72–86. doi:10.5539/gjhs.v4n3p72

14. Konno N, Makita H, Yuri K, Iizuk N, Kawasaki K. Association between Dietary Iodine Intake and Prevalence of Subclinical Hypothyroidism in the Coastal Regions of Japan. *J Clin Endocrinol Metab.* 1994;78(2):393–397. doi:10.1210/jcem.78.2.8106628

15. Eliason BC. Transient Hyperthyroidism in a Patient Taking Dietary Supplements Containing Kelp. *J Am Board Fam Med.* 1998;11(6):478–480. doi:10.3122/jabfm.11.6.478

16. Müssig K, Thamer C, Bares R, Lipp HP, Häring HU, Gallwitz B. Iodine-Induced Thyrotoxicosis after Ingestion of Kelp-Containing Tea. *J Gen Intern Med.* 2006;21(6):c11–c14.

17. Hwang YO, Park SG, Park GY, Choi SM, Kim MY. Total Arsenic, Mercury, Lead, and Cadmium Contents in Edible Dried Seaweed in Korea. *Food Addit Contam Part B Surveill.* 2010;3(1):7–13. doi:10.1080/19440040903532079

18. Michikawa T, Inoue M, Shimazu T, et al. Seaweed Consumption and the Risk of Thyroid Cancer in Women. *Eur J Cancer Prev.* 2012;21(3):254–260. doi:10.1097/CEJ.0b013e32834a8042

19. Food Standards. Advice on Brown Seaweed for Pregnant Women; Breastfeeding Women and Children. Food Standards.

20. FAQs. Selina Naturally. www.selinanaturally.com/faqs. Accessed August 4, 2019.

21. The Importance of Himalayan Pink Salt Iodine and Selenium for Human Body. Himalayan Salt USA. https://himalayansaltusa.com/The-importance-of-Himalayan-Pink-Salt-Iodine-and-Selenium-for-human-body.html. Accessed August 4, 2019.

22. American Heart Association. Study: 70 Percent of Sodium Intake Comes from Restaurant, Processed Foods. American Heart Association News. May 8, 2017.

23. Povidone-Iodine. Wikipedia. https://en.wikipedia.org/wiki/Povidone-iodine. Accessed September 12, 2019.

24. PVP [product page]. Making Cosmetics. https://www.makingcosmetics.com/PVP_p_313.html. Accessed August 4, 2019.

25. Huangshan Bonsun Pharmacuticals. Application of PVP in Daily Chemical Industry. http://www.nhpvp.com/pvp_detai_en/id/35.html. Accesssed September 10, 2019.

26. Nobukuni K, Hayakawa N, Namba R, et al. The Influence of Long-Term Treatment with Povidone-Iodine on Thyroid Function. *Dermatology.* 1997;195:69–72. doi:10.1159/000246034

27. Findik RB, Yilmaz G, Celik HT, Yilmaz FM, Hamurcu U, Karakaya J. Effect of Povidone Iodine on Thyroid Functions and Urine Iodine Levels in Caesarean Operations. *J Matern Neonatal Med.* 2014;27(10):1020–1022. doi:10.3109/14767058.2013.847417

28. Arena Ansotegui J, Emparanza Knörr J, San Millán Vege M, Garrido Chércoles A, Eguileor Gurtubai I. Iodine Overload in Newborn Infants Caused by the Use of PVP-Iodine for Perineal Preparation of the Mother in Vaginal Delivery. *An Españoles Pediatría.* 1989;30(1):23–26.

29. Erdoğan MF, Tatar FA, Ünlütürk U, Cin N, Uysal AR. The Effect of Scrubbing Hands with Iodine-Containing Solutions on Urinary Iodine Concentrations of the Operating Room Staff. *Thyroid.* 2013;23(3):342–345. doi:10.1089/thy.2012.0325

30. Ibid.

31. Nesvadbova M, Crosera M, Maina G, Filon FL. Povidone Iodine Skin Absorption: An Ex-Vivo Study. *Toxicol Lett.* 2015;235(3):155–160. doi:10.1016/j.toxlet.2015.04.004

32. Food and Drug Administration; HHS. Safety and Effectiveness of Consumer Antiseptics; Topical Antimicrobial Drug Products for Over-the-Counter Human Use. *Dly J United States Gov.* 2016;81(172):1–25.

33. Tomoda C, Kitano H, Uruno T, et al. Transcutaneous Iodine Absorption in Adult Patients with Thyroid Cancer Disinfected with Povidone–Iodine at Operation. *Thyroid.* 2005;15(6):600–603. doi:10.1089/thy.2005.15.600

34. Mahillon J, Peers W, Bourdoux P, Ermans AM, Delange F. Effect of Vaginal Douching with Povidone-Iodine during Early Pregnancy on the Iodine Supply to Mother and Fetus. *Biol Neonate.* 1989;56:210–217. doi:10.1159/000243125

35. Allain P, Berre S, Krari N, et al. Use of Plasma Iodine Assay for Diagnosing Thyroid. *J Clin Pathol.* 1993;28(2020):453–455.

36. Cowling T, Frey N. *Macrocyclic and Linear Gadolinium Based Contrast Agents for Adults Undergoing Magnetic Resonance Imaging: A Review of Safety.* Ottawa: Canadian Agency for Drugs and Technologies in Health, 2019.

37. Leung AM, Pearce EN, Braverman LE. Iodine Content of Prenatal Multivitamins in the United States. *N Engl J Med.* 2009;360(9):939–940. doi:10.1056/NEJMc0807851

CHAPTER FIVE

1. Brabant G, Prank K, Ranft U, et al. Physiological Regulation of Circadian and Pulsatile Thyrotropin Secretion in Normal Man and Woman. *J Clin Endocrinol Metab.* 1990;70(2):403–409. doi:10.1210/jcem-70-2-403

2. Mahadevan S, Sadacharan D, Kannan S, Suryanarayanan A. Does Time of Sampling or Food Intake Alter Thyroid Function Test? *Indian J Endocrinol Metab.* 2017;21(3):369–372. doi:10.4103/ijem.IJEM_15_17

3. Kamat V, Hecht WL, Rubin RT. Influence of Meal Composition on the Postprandial Response of the Pituitary-Thyroid Axis. *Eur J Endocrinol.* 1995;133(1):75–79. doi:10.1530/eje.0.1330075

4. Bajaña W, Aranda E, Arredondo M, et al. Impact of an Andean Breakfast on Biochemistry and Immunochemistry Laboratory Tests: An Evaluation on Behalf COLABIOCLI WG-PRE-LATAM. *Biochem Medica.* 2019;29(2):020702. doi:10.11613/BM.2019.020702.

5. Roelfsema F, Johannes D. Thyrotropin Secretion Patterns in Health and Disease. *Endocr Rev.* 2013;34(5):619–657. doi:10.1210/er.2012–1076

6. Tanguay M, Girard J, Scarsi C, Mautone G, Larouche R. Pharmacokinetics and Comparative Bioavailability of a Levothyroxine Sodium Oral Solution and Soft Capsule. *Clin Pharmacol Drug Dev.* 2018;8(13):1–8. doi:10.1002/cpdd.608

7. Kahn K. Iodine Content of Fast Foods Contributes Little to Iodine Levels in the Body. *Medscape.* 4.28.2010. https://www.medscape.com/viewarticle/720930

8. Benvenga S, Di Bari F, Granese R, Antonelli A. Serum Thyrotropin and Phase of the Menstrual Cycle. *Front Endocrinol (Lausanne).* 2017;8:250. doi:10.3389/fendo.2017.00250

9. Benvenga S, Di Bari F, Granese R, et al. Circulating Thyrotropin Is Upregulated by Estradiol. *J Clin Transl Endocrinol.* 2018;11:11–17. doi:10.1016/j.jcte.2018.02.002

10. U.S. Food and Drug Administration. *Total Diet Study: Elements Results Summary Statistics—Market Baskets 2006 through 2013.* USDA, 2014.

11. Mason R. Chlorella and Spirulina: Green Supplements for Balancing the Body. *Altern Complement Ther.* June 2001:28(2020): 161–165. National Institutes of Health. Iodine: Fact Sheet for Health Professionals. NIH. May 1, 2010.

12. Teas J, Pino S, Critchley AT, Braverman LE. Variability of Iodine Content in Common Commercially Available Edible Seaweeds. *Thyroid.* 2004;14(10):836–841. doi:10.1089/thy.2004.14.836

13. Matana A, Torlak V, Brdar D, et al. Dietary Factors Associated with Plasma Thyroid Peroxidase and Thyroglobulin Antibodies. *Nutrients.* 2017;9(11):1186. doi:10.3390/nu9111186

14. Barcza Stockler-Pinto M, Carrero J, De Carvalho Cardoso Weide L, Franciscato Cozzolino S, Mafra D. Effect of Selenium Supplementation via Brazil Nut (Bertholletia Excelsa, HBK) on Thyroid Hormones Levels in Hemodialysis Patients: A Pilot Study. *Nutr Hosp.* 2015;32(4):1808–1812. doi:10.3305/nh.2015.32.4.9384

15. Martens IBG, Cardoso BR, Hare DJ, et al. Selenium Status in Preschool Children Receiving a Brazil Nut–Enriched Diet. *Nutrition.* 2015;31(11):1339–1343. doi:10.1016/j.nut.2015.05.005

16. Kaličanin D, Brčić L, Ljubetić K, Barić A, Gračan S, Brekalo M, Torlak Lovrić V, Kolčić I, Polašek O, Zemunik T, Punda A, Boraska Perica V. Differences in food consumption between patients with Hashimoto's thyroiditis and healthy individuals. *Sci Rep.* 2020 Jun 30;10(1):10670. doi: 10.1038/s41598-020-67719-7. PMID: 32606353; PMCID: PMC7327046

17. Danforth E, Horton ES, O'Connell M, et al. dietary-Induced Alterations in Thyroid Hormone Metabolism during Overnutrition. *J Clin Invest.* 1979;64(5):1336–1347. doi:10.1172/JCI109590

18. Bisschop PH, Sauerwein HP, Endert E, Romijn JA. Isocaloric Carbohydrate Deprivation Induces Protein Catabolism Despite a Low T3-Syndrome in Healthy Men. *Clin Endocrinol (Oxf)*. 2001;54(1):75–80. doi:10.1046/j.1365–2265.2001.01158.x

19. Serog P, Apfelbaum M, Autissier N, Baigts F, Brigant L, Ktorza A. Effects of Slimming and Composition of Diets on VO2 and Thyroid Hormones in Healthy Subjects. *Am J Clin Nutr*. 1982;35(1):24–35. doi:10.1093/ajcn/35.1.24

20. Spaulding SW, Chopra IJ, Sherwin RS, Lyall SS. Effect of Caloric Restriction and Dietary Composition of Serum T3 and Reverse T3 in Man. *J Clin Endocrinol Metab*. 1976;42(1):197–200. doi:10.1210/jcem-42-1-197

21. Pałkowska-Goździk E, Lachowicz K, Rosołowska-Huszcz D. Effects of Dietary Protein on Thyroid Axis Activity. *Nutrients*. 2018;10(1):5.

22. Barrows K, Snook JT. Effect of a High-Protein, Very-Low-Calorie Diet on Resting Metabolism, Thyroid Hormones, and Energy Expenditure of Obese Middle-Aged Women. *Am J Clin Nutr*. 1987;45(2):391–398. doi:10.1093/ajcn/45.2.391

23. Gardner CD, Trepanowski JF, Del Gobbo LC, et al. Effect of Low-Fat vs Low-Carbohydrate Diet on 12-Month Weight Loss in Overweight Adults and the Association with Genotype Pattern or Insulin Secretion. *JAMA*. 2018;319(7):667–679. doi:10.1001/jama.2018.0245

24. Nacamulli D, Mian C, Petricca D, et al. Influence of Physiological Dietary Selenium Supplementation on the Natural Course of Autoimmune Thyroiditis. *Clin Endocrinol (Oxf)*. 2010;73(4):535–539. doi:10.1111/j.1365-2265.2009.03758.x

25. Shreenath AP, Dooley J. *Selenium Deficiency*. Treasure Island, FL: StatPearls, 2020.

26. MacFarquhar J, Broussard D, Melstrom P, et al. Acute Selenium Toxicity Associated with a Dietary Supplement. *Arch Intern Med*. 2010;170(3):256–261.

27. Luo J, Hendryx M, Dinh P, He. K. Association of Iodine and Iron with Thyroid Function. *Biol Trace Elem Res*. 2017;179(1):38–44. doi:10.1007/s12011-017-0954-x

28. Aihara K, Nishi Y, Hatano S, et al. Zinc, Copper, Manganese, and Selenium Metabolism in Thyroid Disease. *Am J Clin Nutr*. 1984;40(1):26–35.

29. Mahmoodianfard S, Vafa M, Golgiri F, et al. Effects of Zinc and Selenium Supplementation on Thyroid Function in Overweight and Obese Hypothyroid Female Patients: A Randomized Double-Blind Controlled Trial. *J Am Coll Nutr*. 2015;34(5):391–399. doi:10.1080/07315724.2014.926161

30. Silva N, Santos O, Morais F, et al. Subclinical Hypothyroidism Represents an Additional Risk Factor for Coronary Artery Calcification, Especially in Subjects with Intermediate and High Cardiovascular Risk Scores. *Eur J Endocrinol*. 2014;171(3):327–334. doi:10.1530/EJE-14-0031

31. Meuwese CL, Olauson H, Qureshi AR, et al. Associations between Thyroid Hormones, Calcification Inhibitor Levels and Vascular Calcification in End-Stage Renal Disease. *PLoS One*. 2015;10(7):e0132353. doi:10.1371/journal.pone.0132353
32. WHO. Population Nutrient Intake Goals for Preventing Diet-Related Chronic Diseases. World Health Organization. https://www.who.int/nutrition/topics/5_population_nutrient/en/. Accessed 8.4.2019.
33. Harvard Women's Health Watch. How Much Calcium Do You Really Need? Harvard Health Publishing. 9.11.2018. https://www.health.harvard.edu/staying-healthy/how-much-calcium-do-you-really-need
34. Leung AM, Lamar A, He X, Braverman LE, Pearce EN. Iodine Status and Thyroid Function of Boston–area Vegetarians and Vegans. *J Clin Endocrinol Metab*. 2011;96(8):e1303–e1307. doi:10.1210/jc.2011-0256
35. Tonstad S, Nathan E, Oda K, Fraser G. Vegan Diets and Hypothyroidism. *Nutrients*. 2013;5(11):4642–4652. doi:10.3390/nu5114642

CHAPTER SIX

1. Hall KD, et al. Ultra-Processed Diets Cause Excess Calorie Intake and Weight Gain: A One-Month Inpatient Randomized Controlled Trial of Ad Libitum Food Intake. *Cell Metab*. 2019;30(1):67-87. doi:10.1016/j.cmet.2019.05.008
2. Rauber F, da Costa Louzada ML, Steele EM, Millett C, Monteiro CA, Levy RB. Ultra-Processed Food Consumption and Chronic Non-Communicable Diseases-Related Dietary Nutrient Profile in the UK (2008-2014). *Nutrients*. 2018;10(5):E587. doi:10.3390/nu10050587
3. Rico-Campà A, Martínez-González MA, Alvarez-Alvarez I, de Deus Mendonça R, de la Fuente-Arrillaga C, Gómez-Donoso C. Association between Consumption of Ultra-Processed Foods and All Cause Mortality: SUN Prospective Cohort Study. *BMJ*. 2019;365:l1949. doi:10.1136/bmj.l1949
4. Fontenelle LC, Feitosa MM, Severo JS, et al. Thyroid Function in Human Obesity: Underlying Mechanisms. *Horm Metab Res*. 2016;48(12):787–794. doi:10.1055/s-0042-121421
5. Kuhs H, Farber D, Tolle R. Serum Prolactin, Growth Hormone, Total Corticoids, Thyroid Hormones, and Thyrotropine During Serial Therapeutic Sleep Deprivation. *Biol Psychiatry*. 1996;39(10):857–864. doi:10.1016/0006-3223(95)00240-5
6. Kessler L, Nedeltcheva A, Imperial J, Penev PD. Changes in Serum TSH and Free T4 during Human Sleep Restriction. *Sleep*. 2010;33(8):1115–1118.
7. Baumgartner A, Dietzel M, Saletu B, et al. Influence of Partial Sleep Deprivation on the Secretion of Thyrotropin, Thyroid Hormones, Growth Hormone, Prolactin, Luteinizing Hormone, Follicle Stimulating Hormone, and Estradiol in Healthy Young Women. *Psychiatry Res*. 1993;48(2):153–178. doi:10.1016/0165-1781(93)90039-j

8. Hsiao YH, Chen YT, Tseng CM, et al. Sleep Disorders and Increased Risk of Autoimmune Diseases in Individuals without Sleep Apnea. *Sleep*. 2015;38(4):581–586. doi:10.5665/sleep.4574
9. Young KA, Munroe ME, Harley JB, et al. Less Than Seven Hours of Sleep per Night Is Associated with Transitioning to Systemic Lupus Erythematosus. *Lupus*. 2018;27(9):1524–1531. doi:10.1177/0961203318778368
10. Kang JH, Lin HC. Obstructive Sleep Apnea and the Risk of Autoimmune Diseases: A Longitudinal Population-Based Study. *Sleep Med*. 2012;13(6):583–588. doi:10.1016/j.sleep.2012.03.002
11. Vural EM, van Munster BC, de Rooij SE. Optimal Dosages for Melatonin Supplementation Therapy in Older Adults: A Systematic Review of Current Literature. *Search Results*. 2014;31(6):441–451. doi:10.1007/s40266-014-0178-0
12. Kripke DF, Langer RD, Kline LE. Hypnotics' Association with Mortality or Cancer: A Matched Cohort Study. *BMJ Open*. 2012;21:e000850. doi:10.1136/bmjopen-2012-000850
13. Kim K, Gu MO, Jung JH, et al. Efficacy of a Home–Based Exercise Program after Thyroidectomy for Thyroid Cancer Patients. *Thyroid*. 2018;28(2):236–245. doi:10.1089/thy.2017.0277

CHAPTER SEVEN

1. Rachdaoui N, Sarkar DK. Pathophysiology of the Effects of Alcohol Abuse on the Endocrine System. *Alcohol Res*. 2017;38(2):255–276.
2. Kim SY, Park JM, Hwang JP. Analysis of Iodine Content in Salts and Korean Sauces for Low=Iodine Diet Education in Korean Patients with Thyroid Cancer Preparing for Radioiodine Therapy. *Nucl Med Mol Imaging*. 2018;52(3):229–233. doi:10.1007/s13139-017-0511-8
3. Tanquay M, Girard J, Scarsi C, Mautone G, Larouche R. Pharmacokenetics and Comparative Bioavailability of a Levothyroxine Socium Oral Solution and Soft Capsule. *Clin Pharmacol Drug Dev*. 2018;8(13):1–8. doi:10.1002/cpdd.608
4. Itano A. Investigation on Agar as to Its Iodine Content. *J Agric Chem Soc Japan*. 1933;9(8):398–401.

CHAPTER NINE

1. Sinclair D. Thyroid Antibodies: Which, Why, When, and Who? Editorial. *Expert Rev Clin Immunol*. 2006;2(5):665–669. doi:10.1586/1744666X.2.5.665
2. Mincer DL, Jialal I. *Hashimoto Thyroiditis*. Treasure Island, FL: StatPearls, 2020.
3. Davies TF. Pathogenesis of Hashimoto's Thyroiditis (Chronic Autoimmune Thyroiditis). UpToDate. January 3, 2020. https://www.uptodate.com/contents/pathogenesis-of-hashimotos-thyroiditis-chronic-autoimmune-thyroiditis.

4. Malya FU, Kadioglu H, Hasbahceci M, Dolay K, Guzel M, Ersoy YE. The Correlation between Breast Cancer and Urinary Iodine Excretion Levels. *J Int Med Res.* 2018;46(2):687–692. doi:10.1177/0300060517717535
5. Smyth PP, Shering SG, Kilbane MT, et al. Serum Thyroid Peroxidase Autoantibodies, Thyroid Volume, and Outcome in Breast Carcinoma. *J Clin Endocrinol Metab.* 1998;83(8):2711–2716. doi:10.1210/jcem.83.8.5049
6. Davies TF. Pathogenesis of Hashimoto's Thyroiditis (Chronic Autoimmune Thyroiditis). UpToDate. 1.3.2020. https://www.uptodate.com/contents/pathogenesis-of-hashimotos-thyroiditis-chronic-autoimmune-thyroiditis.
7. Lebwohl B, Cao Y, Zong G, et al. Long Term Gluten Consumption in Adults without Celiac Disease and Risk of Coronary Heart Disease: Prospective Cohort Study. *BMJ.* 2017;357:J1892. doi:10.1136/bmj.j1892
8. Potter EMDE, Brienesse CS, Walker M, Boyle A, Talley N. Effect of the Gluten–Free Diet on Cardiovascular Risk Factors in Patients with Coeliac Disease: A Systematic Review. *J Gastroenterol Hepatol.* 2018;33(4):781–791. doi:10.1111/jgh.14039
9. Sategna-Guidetti C, Volta U, Ciacci C, et al. Prevalence of Thyroid Disorders in Untreated Adult Celiac Disease Patients and Effect of Gluten Withdrawal: An Italian Multicenter Study. *Am J Gastroenterol.* 2001;96(3):751–757. doi:10.1111/j.1572–0241.2001.03617.x
10. Rakeshkumar Sharma B, Joshi AS, Varthakavi PK, Chadha MD, Bhagwat NM, Pawal PS. Celiac Autoimmunity in Autoimmune Thyroid Disease Is Highly Prevalent with a Questionable Impact. *Indian J Endocrinol Metab.* 2016;20(1):97–100.
11. Chartoumpekis DV, Ziros PG, Chen JG, Groopman JD, Kensler TW, Sykiotis GP. Broccoli Sprout Beverage Is Safe for Thyroid Hormonal and Autoimmune Status: Results of a 12-Week Randomized Trial. *Food Chem Toxicol.* 2019;126:1–6. doi:10.1016/j.fct.2019.02.004
12. Bhagwat S, Haytowitz DB, Holden JM. *USDA Database for the Isoflavone: Content of Selected Foods—Release 2.0.* Beltsville, MD: USDA, 2008.
13. Eisenbrand G, Gelbke H-P. Assessing the Potential Impact on the Thyroid Axis of Environmentally Relevant Food Constituents/Contaminants in Humans. *Arch Toxicol.* 2016;90(8):1841–1857. doi:10.1007/s00204-016-1735-6
14. Steinmaus CM. Perchlorate in Water Supplies: Sources, Exposures, and Health Effects. *Curr Environ Heal Reports.* 2016;3(2):136–143. doi:10.1007/s40572-016-0087-y
15. Steinmaus C, Pearl M, Kharrazi M, et al. Thyroid Hormones and Moderate Exposure to Perchlorate during Pregnancy in Women in Southern California. *Environ Health Perspect.* 2016;124(6):861–867. doi:10.1289/ehp.1409614
16. Leung AM, Pearce EN, Braverman LE. Perchlorate, Iodine, and the Thyroid. *Best Pract Res Clin Endocrinol Metab.* 2010;24(1):133–141. doi:10.1016/j.beem.2009.08.009
17. Macht H. Hypothyroidism in Children. EndocrineWeb 1.5.17. https://www.endocrineweb.com/conditions/hypothyroidism/hypothyroidism-children.

18. Kose E, Guzel O, Demir K, Arsian N. Changes of Thyroid Hormonal Status in Patients Receiving Ketogenic Diet Due to Intractable Epilepsy. *J Pediatr Endocrinol Metab.* 2017;30(4):411–416. doi:10.1515/jpem-2016-0281

19. Gilletz N. *The Low Iodine Diet Cookbook*. eBook. n.p.: Your Health Press, 2005.

20. Otun J, Sahebkar A, Östlundh L, Atkin SL, Sathyapalan T. Systematic Review and Meta-Analysis on the Effect of Soy on Thyroid Function. *Sci Rep.* 2019;9(1):1–9. doi:10.1038/s41598-019-40647-x

21. National Toxicology Program. NTP-CERHR Monograph on Soy Infant Formula. *NTP CERHR MON.* 2010;(23):i–661.

22. Ahsan M, Mallick AK. The Effect of Soy Isoflavones on the Menopause Rating Scale Scoring in Perimenopausal and Postmenopausal Women: A Pilot Study. *J Clin Diagnostic Res.* 2017;11(9):FC13–FC16. doi:10.7860/JCDR/2017/26034.10654

23. Sekikawa A, Ihara M, Lopez O, et al. Effect of S-equol and Soy Isoflavones on Heart and Brain. *Curr Cardiol Rev.* 2019;15(2):114–135. doi:10.2174/1573403X15666181205104717

24. Zheng X, Lee S-K, Chun OK. Soy Isoflavones and Osteoporotic Bone Loss: A Review with an Emphasis on Modulation of Bone Remodeling. *J Med Food.* 2016;19(1):1–14. doi:10.1089/jmf.2015.0045

25. Messina M. Impact of Soy Foods on the Development of Breast Cancer and the Prognosis of Breast Cancer Patients. Forsch Komplementmed. 2016;23(2):75–80. doi:10.1159/000444735

26. Gaksch M, Jorde R, Grimnes G, et al. Vitamin D and Mortality: Individual Participant Data Meta-Analysis of Standardized 25-Hydroxyvitamin D in 26916 Individuals from a European Consortium. *PLoS One.* 2017;12(2):e0170791. doi:10.1371/journal.pone.0170791

27. Crescioli C, Minisola S. Vitamin D: Autoimmunity and Gender. *Curr Med Chem.* 2017;24(24):2671–2686. doi:10.2174/0929867323666161220105821

28. Zittermann A, Ernst JB, Prokop S, et al. Effect of Vitamin D on All-Cause Mortality in Heart Failure (EVITA): A 3-Year Randomized Clinical Trial with 4000 IU Vitamin D Daily. *Eur Heart J.* 2017;38(29):2279–2286. doi:10.1093/eurheartj/ehx235

Acknowledgments

The ideas behind this book came from many sources, all of which deserve credit. Here are the main sources listed in the order in which they influenced me.

First, none of this would have been possible without a love of learning. My parents, Glen and Vivian Christianson, helped me learn to read at an early age. They also prioritized education enough to get me my own encyclopedia set.

After starting the practice of medicine, my patients became among my top teachers. Many of them shared with me their experience with iodine. They made me aware of the emergent ideas of the Iodine Project.

Next would be Dr. Guy Abraham. He graciously shared his work and gave freely of his time. Even though my quest led me to reject his conclusions, he was a kind man and made a strong case for his views.

Soon after my time with Dr. Abraham, Dr. Alan Gaby spotlighted the dangers of high-dose iodine. He worked carefully to peel back many of the growing misconceptions. I read his work and corresponded with him about the concepts.

For many years, I was aware of the harm of megadose iodine, but not of the possible benefits of iodine restriction. I had seen some studies suggesting a link between iodine reduction and remission from thyroid disease, but for some reason, I did not pursue it at first.

A few years later, our medical residents found some of the more dramatic studies and highlighted their findings. They and Drs. Raquel Espinol, Linda Khoshaba, and Rosalyn Ranon helped me think through the implications and work through possible flaws in the theory.

Thanks also go to my agents, Celeste Fein and John Maas, and my publishing team, led by Diana Baroni and Michele Eniclerico. These ideas were buried in an overwhelming manuscript covering nearly every facet of thyroid disease. They helped me understand what was truly distinct about this book and give it the focus it deserved.

Finally, this work would not have been possible without spending over twenty hours per week, for nearly a year, with all the medical literature on thyroid disease. I would not have had the ability to work this hard were it not for mentorship and inspiration from J. J. Virgin.

Thanks to you all. I'm excited that this work will ensure that fewer people will suffer from thyroid disease.

Alan Christianson, NMD
Phoenix, AZ 2020

Index

A
alcohol, 128
American Thyroid Association, 20–21, 79
amiodarone, 46, 74
antibodies (thyroid-attacking), 39, 69, 85, 100, 243–44
anti-thyroglobulin (anti-Tg), 39, 85
anti-thyroid peroxidase (anti-TPO), 39, 85
anxiety, 40, 41, 120, 242
Apple and Brazil Nut Cobbler, 240
autoimmune hypothyroidism. *See* Hashimoto's thyroiditis
autoimmune paleo (AIP) diet adaptions, 91, 105–7. *See also specific recipes*

B
baby formulas, 252
baked goods, 62–63, 65–66. *See also* breads
Basic Brown Rice, 228
Basic Greens, 229
beans. *See* legumes
beef. *See* meats and poultry
Better Than Carry-Out Orange Chicken, 220–21
beverages, 128–29. *See also* shakes
Blastocystis hominis, 251
bloating, 39, 41, 242
bowl recipes. *See* salads, bowls and wraps
BPA exposure, 46
Brazil nuts, 97, 100, 159, 160, 176, 178, 240
breads
 commercially baked, 62–63, 65–66
 Easy Flatbread, 95, 226–27
 Healthy Caesar Salad, 182–83
 Whole-Grain Sourdough Bread, 232–33
breakfast recipes. *See also* shakes
 about: ideas for, 157–58; meal assembly, 143–47
 Brazil Nut Quickbread, 176
 Buckwheat Berry Porridge, 171
 Easy Breakfast Oatmeal, 167
 Egg White Omelet, 168
 Huevos Rancheros, 173
 Overnight Apple Pie Oats, 177
 Pecan-Banana Teff Cereal, 174
 Sweet Potato Hash, 170
 Three-Ingredient Pancakes, 169
 Vanilla Millet Hot Cereal, 172
 Whole Oat Porridge, 175
breast cancer, 243–44, 253
breastfeeding, 60, 68
Buckwheat Banana Bread, 178
Buckwheat Berry Porridge, 171

C

cadmium exposure, 46
Cajun Catfish, 222-23
calcium, 102-3
cancer. *See* breast cancer; thyroid cancer
carbohydrates, 98, 99-100, 258
case stories
    on conventional treatment failure, 21-25
    on hair loss, 73-74
    on Hashimoto's thyroiditis, 124-25
    on hyperthyroidism, 54
    invisible iodine sources, 69, 73-74
    on iodine supplementation, 54
    on medical teams, 124-25
    on Thyroid Reset Diet, without hormone use, 30-31
causes of thyroid disease. *See also* goiters; Graves' disease
    autoimmune link, 11, 20, 39, 46. *See also* Hashimoto's thyroiditis
    environmental factors, 46
    existential factors, 45-46, 61
    iodine excess, 27, 38, 46-47, 50-51, 59-62
    parasites, 251
    sleep disorders, 119-20
    studies on, 47-56
    thyroid antibodies, 39, 69, 85, 100, 243-44
    thyroidectomy, 39
    weight gain, 90, 113-14
celiac disease, 244-45
Celtic light gray sea salt, 69-70, 91
Ceviche Salad, 187
Chai Potato Bowl, 184-85
Chermoula Baked River Trout, 115, 225
chicken. *See* meats and poultry
chlorella, 68
chocolate, 159-60, 246, 247
chronic autoimmune hypothyroidism. *See* Hashimoto's thyroiditis
Cilantro Shrimp Bowl, 186
Classic Niçoise Salad, 181
Classic Split Pea Soup, 200
coconut flakes, 169, 175
commercially baked goods, 62-63, 65-66
commercial salts, 69
condiments, 129-30
conditioners, 71, 72
constipation, 40, 41
conventional treatment, 21-25
cosmetics, 71-73, 92, 104
Creamy Tarragon Chicken, 210-11
cryptosporidium, 251

D

Daily Reset Pack, 77, 94, 103
dairy products
    Green Light list, 130
    as invisible iodine sources, 63-66
    during Maintenance phase, 114, 115
    one-week tiered transition from, 92, 95
    Red Light list, 131
    substitutions, 92, 95, 130. *See also* non-dairy products
    Yellow Light list, 131
Denmark, 15, 51-52
depression, 40, 41, 242
desserts, 238-40
diarrhea, 40, 41, 100, 251
dicalcium malate, 103
dietary supplements
    Daily Reset Pack, 77, 94, 103
    iodine content in, 17, 26-27, 76-77
    megadose iodine supplements, 17, 23, 24, 48
    one-week tiered transition for, 93-94
    QuickStart guide for, 104
    vitamin D, 253
dizziness, 23, 40
dough conditioners, 63
Dr. Khoshaba's Lentil Soup, 195

E

Easy Breakfast Oatmeal, 115, 167
Easy Flatbread, 95
eggs
    about: iodine levels in, 28, 66-67
    boiled eggs, 181
    Green Light list, 131
    during Maintenance phase, 114
    Red Light list, 131
    substitutions, 92, 95. *See also* egg whites
    Yellow Light list, 131
    yolks, 66, 114, 115
egg whites
    about: substitute equivalent measure, 95; as whole egg substitute, 67, 92

INDEX | 279

Brazil Nut Quickbread, 176
Classic Niçoise Salad, 181
Egg White Omelet, 168
Huevos Rancheros, 173
Protein Shake Basic Recipe, 144
Skillet Dish Basic Recipe, 146–47
Sweet Potato Hash, 170
Three-Ingredient Pancakes, 169
Entamoeba histolytica, 251
epidemiologic studies, 47, 50–54
exercise, 120

F

facial moisturizers, 71–72
fatigue
  case stories, 21–25, 30–31
  causes, 41, 100, 242
  thyroid disease symptom, 27–28, 39, 40
fats, 97, 99–100, 258
fermented foods, 133
fertility issues, 41
fibrotic breast disease, 52–53
15-Bean Soup, 198
fish. *See* seafood and fish
flatbread, 92, 95
flours. *See* breads; grains
Flower of the Ocean salt, 69–70
fluid retention, 34, 40
folic acid, 94
Food and Drug Administration (FDA), 26, 63–68, 71, 89
forgetfulness, 27–28, 40
Freekeh Tabbouleh, 179
fruits
  about: Green Light list, 132; polyphenols in, 246; Red Light list, 133; Yellow Light list, 132–33
  Apple and Brazil Nut Cobbler, 240
  Apple Pie Shake, 166
  Better Than Carry-Out Orange Chicken, 220–21
  Brazil Nut Quickbread, 176
  Buckwheat Banana Bread, 178
  Buckwheat Berry Porridge, 171
  Chicken with Peaches and Black Beans, 216
  Chocolate Cherry Swirl, 159
  Easy Breakfast Oatmeal, 167
  Eggnog for Breakfast, 161
  Freekeh Tabbouleh, 179
  Hot Cereal Basic Recipe, 145
  Norwegian Amaranth Pudding, 238
  Orange Spice Shake, 165
  Overnight Apple Pie Oats, 177
  Pecan-Banana Teff Cereal, 174
  Pistachio Chia Pudding, 239
  Protein Shake Basic Recipe, 144
  Pumpkin Pie Delight, 164
  Shiitake Soba Bowl, 188
  Three-Ingredient Pancakes, 169
  Vanilla Millet Hot Cereal, 172

G

garlic, 96, 235
Garlic-Lime Calamari, 224
Giardia lamblia, 251
Gingered Tempeh and Broccoli, 212
glucosinolates, 245–46
gluten-free diet, 92, 244–45. *See also specific recipes*
goiters, 38, 50, 52, 59, 252
goitrogens, 245–48
grains
  about: commercial baked goods, 62–63, 65–66; Green Light list, 134; nutritional profile, 98; one-week tiered transition, 92, 95; Red Light list, 134–35; Yellow Light list, 134
  Apple and Brazil Nut Cobbler, 240
  Apple Pie Shake, 166
  Basic Brown Rice, 228
  Brazil Nut Quickbread, 176
  Buckwheat Banana Bread, 178
  Buckwheat Berry Porridge, 171
  Dr. Khoshaba's Lentil Soup, 195
  Easy Breakfast Oatmeal, 167
  Easy Flatbread, 226–27
  Freekeh Tabbouleh, 179
  Homestyle Meatloaf, 204
  Hot Cereal Basic Recipe, 145
  Klubb (Norwegian Potato Dumplings), 230–31
  Minnesota-Style Wild Rice Hot Dish, 207–8
  Norwegian Amaranth Pudding, 238
  Overnight Apple Pie Oats, 177
  Salad Basic Recipe, 148
  Soup Basic Recipe, 149
  Sweet Corn and Sorghum Soup, 194
  Three-Ingredient Pancakes, 169

grains (continued)
  Vanilla Millet Hot Cereal, 172
  Whole-Grain Sourdough Bread, 232–33
  Whole Oat Porridge, 175
Graves' disease, 38, 48, 51–52, 60, 112
green leafy vegetables. See vegetables
Green Light foods
  about, 29, 90
  beverages, 128
  condiments, 129
  dairy products, 130
  eggs, 131
  fermented foods, 133
  fruits, 132
  grains, 134
  herbs and spices, 135
  iodine levels in, 29, 59–60, 81–82
  legumes, 136
  meats and poultry, 137
  nuts and seeds, 138
  seafood and fish, 139–40
  sea vegetables, 141
  vegetables, 141–42
Greens, Alliums, and Cruciferous Veggies, 234

H

hair loss
  case story, 73–74
  causes, 34, 100, 242
  resolution of, 73–74, 83
  thyroid disease symptoms, 27–28, 39, 40
Hashimoto, Hiroko, 11
Hashimoto's thyroiditis
  about, 38–39
  case stories, 21–25, 124–25
  causes, 37, 39, 119
  diagnosis, 39
  invisible iodine sources and, 24
  iodine fortification and, 50–51
  iodine index and, 59–60
  prevalence of, 16, 20, 50–51
  progression of, 39
  reversal of, 12, 13, 27. See also Thyroid Reset Diet
  studies on, 11, 55–56
  thyroid disease cause, 11, 20, 39, 46
  treatment, 22–23
Healthy Caesar Salad, 182–83
herbs and spices, 135–36, 258–59

hidden sources of iodine. See invisible iodine sources
Himalayan salt, 69, 70
Homestyle Beef Stew, 197
Homestyle Meatloaf, 203–4
home thyroid testing, 85
hookworm, 251
hot cereal recipes, 145, 167, 171, 172, 174, 175, 177
Huevos Rancheros, 173
hyperthyroidism
  about, 38
  case story, 54
  causes, 38
  Graves' disease and, 38, 48, 51–52, 60, 112
  iodine-induced, 27, 50–52, 54, 58, 60
  prevalence of, 50
  sea vegetable intake and, 68
  TSH levels and, 36
hyperthyroid storm, 48
hypothyroidism
  about, 38–39
  autoimmune link, 39. See also Hashimoto's thyroiditis
  case story, 30–31
  causes, 27, 39, 45–56. See also causes of thyroid disease
  diagnosis, 36, 39
  iodine index and, 59
  prevalence of, 16, 50–51
  reversal of, 27. See also Thyroid Reset Diet
  symptoms, 35, 39, 40–41

I

insomnia, 38, 40, 119–20, 242
interventional trials, 47, 54–56
invisible iodine sources, 57–70
  about, 19–20, 26
  baked goods, 62–63, 65–66
  case stories, 24–25, 69, 73–74
  cosmetics, 71–73, 92, 104
  dairy products, 63–66
  dietary supplements, 17, 26–27, 76–77
  eating out and, 116–17
  eggs, 28, 66–67
  elimination of, 17–18, 26. See also Thyroid Reset Diet
  fluctuations among, 64, 77–79

INDEX | 281

Hashimoto's thyroiditis and, 24–25
iodine index and, 57–62
medications, 74–76
salt, 15, 25, 26, 69–70
seafood and sea vegetables, 67–69
vaginal douches, 73
iodide, 46
iodine
autoimmune symptoms link, 41, 46, 49
chemical properties of, 26
deficiencies, 13, 15–16, 50, 59
deficiency, 249, 252
hidden sources of, 17, 19–20. *See also* invisible iodine sources
restoring safe levels of, 13–14. *See also* Thyroid Reset Diet
safe range of, 12–13, 16, 18, 46, 52, 249
supplementation, 52–53, 55, 93
testing, 87–88
thyroid disease and, 16–17, 19–20
thyroid function and, 12–13, 18, 26–27, 31, 36–37, 46–47, 48
Wolff Chaikoff effect, 48
iodine index, 57–62
iodine individuality, 88–89
iodine intolerance, 88–89
ionizing radiation, 46
iron, 77, 101
irritable bowel syndrome (IBS), 39
isoflavones, 246, 247, 252

J
joint pain, 40, 100, 103

K
ketogenic diets, 248–49
Kirin's Slow-Cooker Chicken, 213
Klubb (Norwegian Potato Dumplings), 230–31
kosher salt, 70, 91

L
leafy greens. *See* vegetables
legumes
about: Green Light list, 136; isoflavones in, 247; nutritional profile, 98, 101, 102, 103; Red Light list, 136; in shakes, 157–58; Yellow Light list, 136
Apple Pie Shake, 166
Ceviche Salad, 187
Chicken with Peaches and Black Beans, 216
Chocolate Mint Shake, 160
Classic Split Pea Soup, 200
Creamy Lentil Curry, 217–18
Dr. Khoshaba's Lentil Soup, 195
Eggnog for Breakfast, 161
15-Bean Soup, 198
Ginger Spice Shake, 162, 163
Huevos Rancheros, 173
Masala Lentil Wraps, 190–91
Mediterranean Fennel Salad, 180
One-Pot Green Chile Pasta, 215
Orange Spice Shake, 165
Paprika Chicken with Roasted Limas and Brussels Sprouts, 209
Protein Shake Basic Recipe, 144
Roman Wraps, 189
Salad Basic Recipe, 148
Skillet Dish Basic Recipe, 146–47
Soup Basic Recipe, 149
Southwest Scramble Wraps, 193
Thyroid Friendly Pesto, 236
levothyroxine. *See* T4 hormone
lifestyle medicine, 119
liquid egg whites. *See* egg whites
low (metabolism) symptoms, 34–35, 40
low-carbohydrate diet, 98, 99–100
low-iodine diets, 14–15, 19–20, 28, 55–56, 250
lunch and dinner
main courses, 203–25. *See also* main courses
meal assembly for, 148–49
salads, bowls and wraps, 179–93. *See also* salads, bowls and wraps
sides, dressings, and dips, 226–37. *See also* sides, dressings, and dips
soups and stews, 194–202. *See also* soups and stews

M
macronutrients, 97–100, 258
main courses, 203–25
Better Than Carry-Out Orange Chicken, 220–21
Cajun Catfish, 222–23
Chermoula Baked River Trout, 225
Chicken with Peaches and Black Beans, 216

main courses (*continued*)
  Creamy Lentil Curry, 217–18
  Creamy Tarragon Chicken, 210–11
  Garlic-Lime Calamari, 224
  Gingered Tempeh and Broccoli, 212
  Homestyle Meatloaf, 203–4
  Kirin's Slow-Cooker Chicken, 213
  Minnesota-Style Wild Rice Hot Dish, 207–8
  One-Pot Green Chile Pasta, 214–15
  Paprika Chicken with Roasted Limas and Brussels Sprouts, 209
  Poached Garlic Chicken, 219
  Shepherd's Pie, 205–6
Maintenance phase
  about, 84, 111–12, 114–15
  case story, 124–25
  exercise and, 120
  food lists, 127–42. *See also* Green Light foods; Yellow Light foods
  iodine index and, 60
  medical team recommendations, 111–12, 120–25
  restaurant options, 116–18
  sleep and, 119–20
  unprocessed food focus of, 112–14
Masala Lentil Wraps, 190–91
meats and poultry
  about: Green Light list, 137; nutritional profile, 101, 102; Red Light list, 137; Yellow Light list, 137
  Better Than Carry-Out Orange Chicken, 220–21
  Chai Potato Bowl, 184–85
  Chicken with Peaches and Black Beans, 216
  Creamy Lentil Curry, 218
  Creamy Tarragon Chicken, 210–11
  Homestyle Beef Stew, 197
  Homestyle Meatloaf, 203–4
  Kirin's Slow-Cooker Chicken, 213
  Minnesota-Style Wild Rice Hot Dish, 207–8
  One-Pot Green Chile Pasta, 214–15
  Paprika Chicken with Roasted Limas and Brussels Sprouts, 209
  Poached Garlic Chicken, 219
  Roman Wraps, 189
  Salad Basic Recipe, 148
  Sesame Ginger Lettuce Wraps, 192
  Shepherd's Pie, 205–6
  Shiitake Soba Bowl, 188
  Skillet Dish Basic Recipe, 146–47
  Soup Basic Recipe, 149
  Sweet Corn and Sorghum Soup, 194
  Sweet Potato Hash, 170
  White Bean Chile Verde, 196
medical team recommendations, 111–12, 120–25
medications
  iodine content in, 69–70, 74–76
  QuickStart guide for, 104
  for thyroid disease, 22–27, 83–84, 104, 123
Mediterranean Fennel Salad, 115, 180
megadose iodine supplements, 93
memory issues, 27–28, 40
menstrual cycle, 35, 39, 40–41, 101
mercury, 46
metabolic symptoms, 34–35, 40
milk, 63–65, 114. *See also* dairy products; non-dairy products
Minnesota-Style Wild Rice Hot Dish, 207–8
mood swings, 35, 40, 41
multivitamins. *See* dietary supplements
muscle mass loss, 98, 99, 157
muscle pain and cramps, 28, 35, 39, 40
mushrooms
  about, 102
  Creamy Tarragon Chicken, 210–11
  Egg White Omelet, 168
  Minnesota-Style Wild Rice Hot Dish, 207–8
  Shepherd's Pie, 205–6
  Shiitake Soba Bowl, 188

N

nails, brittle and ridged, 35, 40
Niçoise salad, 181
non-dairy products, 65, 92, 95, 130
Norwegian Amaranth Pudding, 238
Norwegian Potato Dumplings (Klubb), 230–31
nuts and seeds
  about: food lists, 138; isoflavones in, 246, 247; nutritional profile, 102, 103
  Apple and Brazil Nut Cobbler, 240
  Apple Pie Shake, 166

Brazil Nut Quickbread, 176
Buckwheat Banana Bread, 178
Buckwheat Berry Porridge, 171
Ceviche Salad, 187
Chocolate Cherry Swirl, 159
Easy Breakfast Oatmeal, 167
Eggnog for Breakfast, 161
Freekeh Tabbouleh, 179
Ginger Spice Shake, 163
Overnight Apple Pie Oats, 177
Pecan-Banana Teff Cereal, 174
Pistachio Chia Pudding, 239
Vanilla Millet Hot Cereal, 172
Whole Oat Porridge, 175

O
obstructive sleep apnea, 119
olives, 180, 181
One-Pot Green Chile Pasta, 115, 214–15
one-week tiered transition, 91–95
osteoporosis, 103
Overnight Apple Pie Oats, 177

P
palpitations, 38, 41, 54
Paprika Chicken with Roasted Limas and Brussels Sprouts, 209
parasites, 251
patient stories. See case stories
Pecan-Banana Teff Cereal, 174
pediatric goiter, 50, 59
perchlorate, 246, 247–48
personal-care products, 71–73
Pico de Gallo, 237
pinworm, 251
Pistachio Chia Pudding, 239
pituitary gland, 36, 119
PMS, 35, 40
Poached Garlic Chicken, 219
polyphenols, 245–46, 247
polyvinylpyrrolidone (PVP), 71
population studies, 47, 50–54
poultry. See meats and poultry
pregnancy, 60, 61, 68
produce. See vegetables
protein powder options, 157–58. See also shakes
proteins, 99, 258
Protein Shake Basic Recipe, 144
psychosis, 41

R
racing heart, 38, 41, 54
radiology contrast agents, 75
Red Light foods
about, 29, 91
beverages, 128
condiments, 130
dairy products, 131
eggs, 132
fermented foods, 133
fruits, 133
grains, 134–35
herbs and spices, 136
iodine index and, 60, 61–62
iodine levels in, 29, 82
legumes, 136
meats and poultry, 137
nuts and seeds, 138
seafood and fish, 140
sea vegetables, 141
vegetables, 141–42
Reset phase
about overview and summary, 82–84
duration of, 83–84
food lists, 127–42. See also Green Light foods
iodine index level for, 59
thyroid medication adjustment during, 83–84
Roasted Garlic, 235
Roman Wraps, 189

S
salads, bowls and wraps
Chai Potato Bowl, 184–85
Cilantro Shrimp Bowl, 186
Classic Niçoise Salad, 181
Freekeh Tabbouleh, 179
Healthy Caesar Salad, 182–83
Masala Lentil Wraps, 190–91
Mediterranean Fennel Salad, 180
Roman Wraps, 189
Salad Basic Recipe, 148
Sesame Ginger Lettuce Wraps, 192
Shiitake Soba Bowl, 188
Southwest Scramble Wraps, 193
salt
bring your own, 116, 138–39
iodine content in, 15, 25, 26, 69–70
options, 69–70, 91–92, 138–39

seafood and fish
  about: Green Light list, 139–40; iodine content in, 67; during Maintenance phase, 115; Red Light list, 140; Yellow Light list, 140
  Cajun Catfish, 222–23
  Calamari Stew, 202
  Ceviche Salad, 187
  Chermoula Baked River Trout, 225
  Cilantro Shrimp Bowl, 186
  food lists, 139–40
  Garlic-Lime Calamari, 224
  Healthy Caesar Salad, 182–83
  Salad Basic Recipe, 148
sea salt, 69, 91–92
sea vegetables, 67–69, 141
seeds. *See* nuts and seeds
selenium, 89, 97, 100
selenomethionine, 97
serving sizes, 90, 128
shakes, 157–66
  about, 157–58
  Apple Pie Shake, 166
  Chocolate Cherry Swirl, 159
  Chocolate Mint Shake, 160
  Eggnog for Breakfast, 161
  Ginger Spice Shake, 162
  Orange Spice Shake, 165
  Peppermint Nut Butter Shake, 163
  Protein Shake Basic Recipe, 144
  Pumpkin Pie Delight, 164
shampoos, 71, 72
Shepherd's Pie, 205–6
Shiitake Soba Bowl, 188. *See also* mushrooms
shopping lists, 257–62
sides, dressings, and dips, 226–37
  Basic Brown Rice, 228
  Basic Greens, 229
  Easy Flatbread, 226–27
  Greens, Alliums, and Cruciferous Veggies, 234
  Klubb (Norwegian Potato Dumplings), 230–31
  Pico de Gallo, 237
  Roasted Garlic, 235
  Thyroid Friendly Pesto, 236
  Whole-Grain Sourdough Bread, 232–33
Skillet Dish Basic Recipe, 146–47
skincare products, 71–73, 92, 104

sleep issues, 38, 40, 119–20, 242
Smart Balance spread, 92
soups and stews, 194–202
  Calamari Stew, 202
  Classic Split Pea Soup, 200
  Curried Kabocha Soup, 201
  Dr. Khoshaba's Lentil Soup, 195
  15-Bean Soup, 198
  Homestyle Beef Stew, 197
  Soup Basic Recipe, 149
  Soup of the Green Goddess, 199
  Sweet Corn and Sorghum Soup, 194
  White Bean Chile Verde, 196
Southwest Scramble Wraps, 193
soy, 246, 247, 252–53
spices and herbs, 135–36, 258–59
spirulina, 68
sunscreens, 71
supplements. *See* dietary supplements
swallowing difficulties, 39, 40
Sweet Corn and Sorghum Soup, 194
Sweet Potato Hash, 115, 170

T
T3 hormone (triiodothyronine)
  about, 35, 37, 85
  carbohydrates and, 98
  carbohydrates' effect on, 98
  exercise and, 120
  in natural desiccated thyroid medication, 123
  sleep and, 119
  as thyroid disease treatment, 23
T4 hormone (levothyroxine)
  about, 35, 37, 85
  hypothyroidism diagnosis and, 39, 85
  in natural desiccated thyroid medication, 123
  sleep's effect on, 119
  as thyroid disease treatment, 22
tea, 245–46
telemedicine, 119, 124–25
tempeh, 101
test tube studies, 47, 48–49
Three-Ingredient Pancakes, 115, 169
thyroglobulin (Tg), 36, 37, 49, 85
thyroid
  anatomy, 33–34
  iodine levels and function of, 12–15, 18, 26–27, 31, 36–37, 46–47, 48

physiology, 34
resiliency of, 31
stimulation of, 36
testing, 28, 29, 84–87, 112, 124
thyroid hormone function, 34–37
thyroid hormone production, 27, 31, 37–39, 46–47
thyroid hormone types, 35–37. *See also* T3 hormone (triiodothyronine); T4 hormone (levothyroxine); thyroid stimulating hormone (TSH)

thyroid cancer
causes, 16–17, 38, 68
prevalence of, 20
screening for, 123–24
TSH levels and, 85

thyroid diets
low-iodine diets, 14–15, 19–20, 28, 55–56, 250–51
Thyroid Reset Diet comparison, 28–29, 250–51. *See also* Thyroid Reset Diet

thyroid disease. *See also* Hashimoto's thyroiditis; hyperthyroidism; hypothyroidism
causes, 45–56. *See also* causes of thyroid disease
conditions associated with, 242
conventional treatment failures, 20–25
differential diagnosis, 242, 251
gluten and, 244–45
invisible iodine sources and, 24. *See also* invisible iodine sources
low-iodine diets as treatment for, 14–15, 19–20, 28, 55–56, 250–51
medication for, 22–27, 83–84, 104, 123
patient stories. *See* case stories
prevalence of, 14, 15, 16–17, 20
process of, 19, 24, 25, 26–27
remission, 243–44
research on, 11–12
reversal of, 12, 13, 17–18, 27–29, 46–47, 55–56, 59. *See also* Thyroid Reset Diet
symptoms of, 11, 27–28, 40–41
symptom survey, 42–43
testing, 28, 29, 84–87, 112, 124

Thyroid Friendly Pesto, 115, 236
thyroid nodules, 38, 52
thyroid peroxidase (TPO), 37, 39, 100, 243–44
Thyroid Reset Diet, 81–109
about: overview and summary, 13–14, 17–18, 20, 27–29; reset, defined, 19
frequently asked questions, 241–53
Green Light, Yellow Light, and Red Light model, 58, 90–91, 128–42. *See also* Green Light foods; Red Light foods; Yellow Light foods
how it works, 29–31
implementation of, 81–82
macronutrients and, 97–100
meal assembly for, 143–49
menu plan, 152–56
micronutrients and, 100–104
other dietary considerations, 96–97
patient stories. *See* case stories
phases overview, 18, 29–30, 82–84. *See also* Maintenance phase; Reset phase
QuickStart guide, 104
recipes, 151–52
research support for, 47–49
serving sizes, 90, 128
shopping lists, 257–62
special diet adaptions, 91, 105–9
thyroid retesting during, 28, 29, 84–87
transition week, 91–95

thyroid stimulating hormone (TSH), 28, 36, 39, 85, 87
topical iodine products, 71, 75
Total Diet Study (TDS), 26, 63–68, 89
toxic nodular goiter, 38
tremors, 40, 41
triiodothyronine. *See* T3 hormone
trypsin inhibitors, 252

U

ultrasounds, 39, 86, 111–12
unprocessed foods, 112–14
urinary iodine to creatine ratio, 87

V

vaginal douches, 73
Vanilla Millet Hot Cereal, 115, 172
vegan diet adaptions, 91–92, 105, 107–9
vegetables
about: glucosinolates in, 245–46; Green Light list, 141–42; nutritional profile, 98, 101, 102, 103; recommended intake, 96; Red Light list, 142; Yellow Light list, 142

Basic Greens, 229
Better Than Carry-Out Orange Chicken, 220–21
Calamari Stew, 202
Ceviche Salad, 187
Chai Potato Bowl, 184–85
Chicken with Peaches and Black Beans, 216
Chocolate Cherry Swirl, 159
Chocolate Mint Shake, 160
Cilantro Shrimp Bowl, 186
Classic Niçoise Salad, 181
Classic Split Pea Soup, 200
Creamy Lentil Curry, 217–18
Creamy Tarragon Chicken, 210–11
Curried Kabocha Soup, 201
Easy Breakfast Oatmeal, 167
Egg White Omelet, 168
15-Bean Soup, 198
Freekeh Tabbouleh, 179
Gingered Tempeh and Broccoli, 212
Greens, Alliums, and Cruciferous Veggies, 234
Healthy Caesar Salad, 182–83
Homestyle Beef Stew, 197
Huevos Rancheros, 173
Klubb (Norwegian Potato Dumplings), 230–31
Masala Lentil Wraps, 190–91
Mediterranean Fennel Salad, 180
Minnesota-Style Wild Rice Hot Dish, 207–8
One-Pot Green Chile Pasta, 214–15
Overnight Apple Pie Oats, 177
Paprika Chicken with Roasted Limas and Brussels Sprouts, 209
Pico de Gallo, 237
Roman Wraps, 189
Salad Basic Recipe, 148
Sesame Ginger Lettuce Wraps, 192
Shepherd's Pie, 205–6
Shiitake Soba Bowl, 188
Skillet Dish Basic Recipe, 146–47
Soup Basic Recipe, 149
Soup of the Green Goddess, 199
Southwest Scramble Wraps, 193
Sweet Corn and Sorghum Soup, 194
Sweet Potato Hash, 170
White Bean Chile Verde, 196
vitamin D, 253
voice changes (hoarse voice), 39, 40

W

weight gain
    causes, 34, 52, 90, 242
    as thyroid disease cause, 90, 113–14
    thyroid disease symptom, 39, 40, 41, 52
weight-loss resistance, 242
wheat allergy, 244–45
White Bean Chile Verde, 196. *See also* legumes
Whole Oat Porridge, 175
Wolff Chaikoff effect, 48
World Health Organization (WHO), 15–16, 57–62
wrap recipes. *See* salads, bowls and wraps

Y

Yellow Light foods
    about, 29, 90
    beverages, 128
    condiments, 130
    dairy products, 131
    eggs, 131
    fermented foods, 133
    fruits, 132–33
    grains, 134
    herbs and spices, 136
    iodine levels in, 29, 82
    legumes, 136
    Maintenance phase consumption of, 29, 82
    meats and poultry, 137
    nuts and seeds, 138
    Reset phase avoidance of, 29, 82
    seafood and fish, 140
    sea vegetable, 141
    vegetables, 141–42

Z

zinc, 102

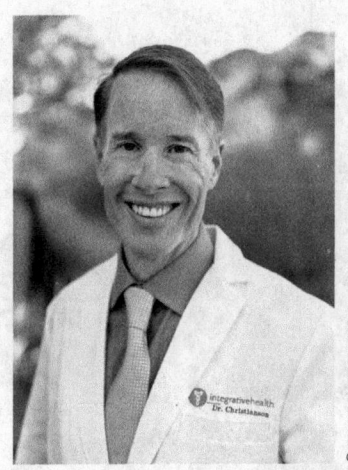

Alan Christianson, NMD, *New York Times* bestselling author of *The Adrenal Reset Diet, The Metabolism Reset Diet, The Thyroid Reset Diet,* and *The Hormone Healing Cookbook,* is a naturopathic medical doctor who specializes in natural endocrinology with a focus on thyroid disorders. He founded Integrative Health, a physician group dedicated to helping people with thyroid disease and weight-loss resistance regain their health. He has been named a Top Doctor in *Phoenix* magazine and has appeared on national TV shows and in print media. Dr. Christianson lives in Phoenix with his wife and their two children.

ALSO BY
ALAN CHRISTIANSON, NMD

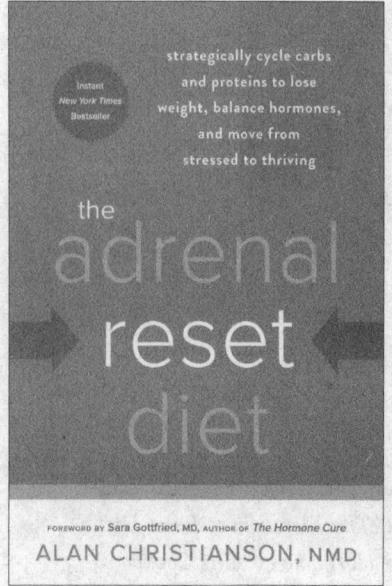
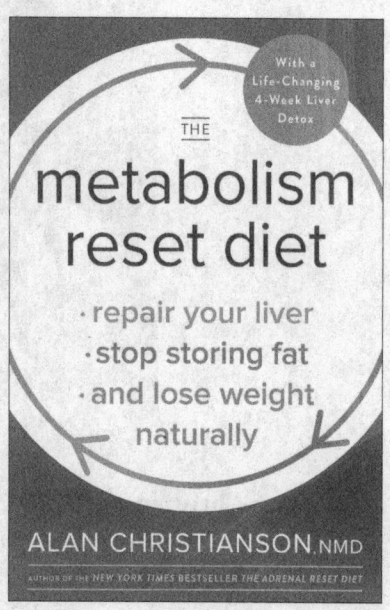

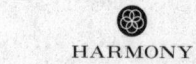
HARMONY
Available wherever books are sold